NUTRIENT-BASED
PSYCHIATRY®

VOLUME 1

NUTRIENT-BASED PSYCHIATRY®

A Nutritional Prescription for ADHD

EMANUEL FRANK, MD
ILLUSTRATIONS BY MAIAH PARDO

ISBN-13: 978-0-9967617-0-3
eISBN: 978-0-9967617-1-0
LCCN: 2016914552

Illustrations by Maiah Pardo

While all of the patient stories described in this book are based on true experiences, all of the names are pseudonyms, and some situations have been changed slightly for educational purposes and to protect each individual's privacy.

The information in this book is not offered, nor should it be used to treat or diagnose any particular disease or any particular patient. Neither the author nor the publisher is engaged in rendering professional advice or services to the individual reader.

For My Family

How to Get the Most from This Book

Patients and parents of children with attention-deficit/hyperactivity disorder (ADHD) should read Part One, which is written in easy-to-understand language for the nonmedical-professional public. Parts Two and Three contain significant scientific details about nutrient-based psychiatry® and different treatment options for those with ADHD. You are encouraged to give the treatment suggestions to your physician(s) and other medical professionals for possible integration into clinical management.

This book is a suggested guide that is compatible with doctor-prescribed stimulant or nonstimulant medications during any phase of treatment. As such, the medical information provided here is *not* a do-it-yourself guide for the treatment of psychiatric disorders, *nor* is it intended or implied to be a substitute for professional medical advice. Always consult your physician or health care provider prior to starting any new treatment or with any questions you may have regarding a medical condition.

Contents

Introduction

Nutrient-Based Psychiatry®, or NBP, is a series of books about using nutritional supplements and dietary modifications to treat psychiatric disorders. Intended to complement conventional psychiatry, this series involves the systematic use of nutritional interventions that may address psychiatric disorders in ways conventional medications do not. This book is Volume 1, which specifically focuses on the treatment of *attention-deficit/ hyperactivity disorder* (ADHD), a disorder characterized by the inability to sustain focus on a task, overactivity (hyperactivity), impulsive behavior, or a combination of these symptoms. ADHD may be influenced by genetic factors, neurochemistry, allergies, and/or environmental and dietary factors; therefore, treatment can be a complex issue. Throughout this book, the term *nutrient-based psychiatry* (or NBP) is also used to refer to the overall approach of using nutrients in the forms of nutritional supplements and dietary modifications as an additional treatment option for ADHD.

Current standard medication management tends to focus on the psychostimulant medications: methylphenidate and amphetamines. Although these medications are effective in most cases, they may also have some adverse effects. Moreover, these interventions may address the symptoms, but they may not address the causes and other complications of the condition. This book aims to educate patients and parents about the role of naturally occurring interventions (meaning dietary changes and nutritional supplements) for ADHD and provide psychiatrists and other prescribing physicians with specific evidence-based treatment strategies designed to be integrated into current clinical practices.

For most physicians, the extent of the discussion in medical school and postdoctoral training about treating diseases with vitamins, minerals, and other nutrients was limited to correcting severe deficiency states. A few psychiatric conditions were included within this category. Throughout my medical training, the notion of treating psychiatric illnesses with natural substances seemed unnecessary to me because we had a variety of effective pharmaceuticals that generally worked well. Then, in 2002, the need to consider nontraditional treatments arose.

At the time, I was working with a client who had a paranoid psychosis. One of the manifestations was suspiciousness of pharmaceutical companies, as well as of doctors. He felt these companies were malevolent entities that were trying to control his thoughts and actions, experiment on him, and possibly trying to poison him with chemicals that had only been in existence for a short time. Therefore, he refused to take anything made by a company that manufactured medications. He was, however, willing to take naturally occurring substances that might help his condition.

He was quite adamant about his beliefs, and I felt my chances of convincing him otherwise were slim. I took a hard look in the medical literature for something that met his requested criteria, which would possibly address his psychotic symptoms. At the time, there was evidence that certain omega-3 fats at the proper dose may have an antipsychotic effect. I presented this information to the client, and he accepted the intervention.

Next, I faced the unexpected difficulty of prescribing a nutritional supplement, which was really a food component and not on the formulary, to a patient in a hospital setting. (Since this time, medical research has found sufficient evidence to create a prescription form of omega-3 fats, which is indicated for elevated triglycerides, and off-label prescribing is possible.) My patient began taking the high-dosage omega-3 fats and, after about two weeks, his suspicions and paranoia seemed to lessen. He also finally agreed that perhaps going back on a prescription antipsychotic medication might be helpful for him, and he did so.

Perhaps the omega-3s had a true antipsychotic or placebo effect that lowered his level of paranoia, thereby allowing him to make the choice to take the necessary antipsychotic prescription medication. It is also possible that my willingness, as his psychiatrist, to work within his parameters built trust and rapport in the doctor-client relationship to the degree that he was willing to accept the medication prescribed *by me.* In any case, this experience gave me pause, and I began to wonder what other nutritional approaches could be used to treat psychiatric disorders. Consequently, and throughout my medical training, I chose to research treating various psychiatric illnesses with nutritional interventions whenever I had the opportunity. In doing so, I was slowly building a knowledge base that I would later integrate into my own psychiatric practice.

I have been practicing child, adolescent, and adult psychiatry in the San Francisco Bay area since 2004. During this time, I have developed a subspecialty that uses nutritional and supplement interventions integrated with psychotherapy and prescription medications. Results have been positive, and I receive more referrals than I can personally accept; it has been difficult to find other psychiatrists with experience in this nutrition-based approach. I have regrettably found myself having to turn away people who could very well have been helped by nutritional interventions.

Prescription medication management in psychiatry, especially child psychiatry, is a highly complex and specialized skill. Many supplements that can be used in treating psychiatric conditions have powerful pharmaceutical effects. It follows that psychiatrists are in a unique position to administer and monitor natural medicines for mental health applications, particularly when integrated with prescription medications and when *comorbid* (the presence of one or more additional disorders that co-occur with the primary disorder) health conditions are present. A growing demand for a natural, *nutrient-based* psychiatric approach and the lack of psychiatrists in this field have created a relative void in current psychiatric practice. Other types of health care professionals do have extensive knowledge of nutrient-based approaches, including medical doctors, nutritionists, and chiropractors. However, this expertise among these professionals and psychiatrists is underrepresented in the clinical community.

A colleague once asked me to give a presentation at his neuropsychiatric clinic about how I had been integrating supplements and dietary management into my practice. While poring over the medical literature in preparation for the talk, I found a sharp increase in the amount of information available in support of nutrient-based approaches for the treatment of mood, anxiety, psychotic, substance abuse, developmental, and other types of psychiatric disorders. This new material included many well-designed studies and meta-analyses.

I informed my colleague that it would take me several months to prepare a lecture summarizing this approach. I realized it was possible to develop specific integrative treatment strategies for many psychiatric disorders on the basis of a medical model that could be used by psychiatrists. This is how the concept of *nutrient-based psychiatry* (NBP), as an integrative psychiatric approach to treating mental illnesses, was born.

It became clear that an NBP text, speaking to parents and patients, as well as clinicians, would be a useful tool for increasing the accessibility of this relevant information to parties on both sides of the equation. I began my research with a focus on ADHD and planned to release a book addressing many psychiatric disorders when all of the chapters on major psychiatric diagnoses and symptoms were complete. However, in order to make this information available in a more timely fashion, I decided to release the ADHD information as the first volume in a series of books on the topic of NBP, which would be published on an ongoing basis.

PART ONE: UNDERSTANDING NUTRIENT-BASED PSYCHIATRY® (NPB)

Part One of this book is primarily written for adults and the parents of children with ADHD. Because treating ADHD with nutrients and dietary modifications is a new concept for many, it is important to understand how it works and why it may be a good option for you or your child. Again, this book is *not* intended to be a do-it-yourself guide, but rather a guide to supplemental or alternative treatment methods to be considered by your medical professionals.

CHAPTER 1

Psychiatry and Conventional Treatment

The human body is a highly complex system that is generally regulated by the brain through the release of chemicals having cascades of effects throughout the body which keep it functioning properly. As with any automated system, there is some amount of wear and tear that occurs with use. Our bodies require certain substances from the environment in order to function, including water, oxygen, amino acids and certain fats, carbohydrates, and vitamins and minerals.

The human body is such a complicated system that, inevitably, things will go wrong. Interdependent factors, such as genetic mutation, lack of essential materials, exposure to toxins, injuries, environmental forces, and aging, can manifest as illness or disease. Mental disorders arise when this pathology affects brain function. *Psychiatry* is the medical specialty that diagnoses and treats mental illness. The treatment of mental disorders has often involved the use of various forms of psychotherapies and medications.

Psychotropic Medications

Psychiatrists are uniquely trained to prescribe and monitor *psychotropic* (those affecting the mind) medications. These are chemicals with powerful effects on brain *neurochemistry*, which is the chemical makeup and activities of nervous tissue (the spinal cord, brain, and nerves). The basic cell of nervous tissue is called a *neuron*. An understanding of the brain, which is the most complex organ in the body, is necessary to grasp the implications of manipulating its functions in any way. (More specific information on this topic is found in later chapters.)

Psychotropic medications have profound effects on mood, behavior, and cognition (thinking), and they can improve the quality of life for those suffering from mental illnesses. In some instances, however, they may be only partially effective or ineffective and may produce unwanted side effects. A growing group of patients does not want to use psychotropic medications for reasons such as these.

In the world of modern medicine, aspiring and established physicians are constantly flooded with pharmaceutical companies' advertising and salespeople, promoting the virtues of their medications in myriad forms. In their medical training, most psychiatrists legitimately devote much time to the proper use of psychotropic medications, which are commonly beneficial and improve the quality of clients' lives, while nutritional considerations are a minor focus.

Prescription medications can be tremendously effective for many medical and psychiatric conditions, but when they are used without considering other safe and effective interventions, they do not provide clients with integrated care.

Newer, Integrative Treatment Options

Nutrient-based psychiatry (NBP) is an integrative psychiatric approach to treating mental illnesses: It is intended to complement conventional psychiatric treatments and involves systematic nutritional interventions. These interventions may address psychiatric disorders in ways conventional medications do not and have fewer (or no) adverse side effects.

In many cases, doctors may consider prescribing nutritional interventions, but only after traditional psychotropic medications don't provide enough relief or produce negative side effects. All too often, treatment becomes fragmented among the doctor's prescription medication approach and other nonmedical providers addressing nutritional and supplement issues. The relative lack of knowledge about each other's disciplines is not optimal for patient care.

Several factors have created the need for a well-researched and systematic guide for integrating nutritional interventions into

4

psychiatry. Over many years of adding nutritional approaches into my own psychiatric practice, I have observed positive results in treating a variety of psychiatric conditions—including mood, anxiety, psychotic, developmental, cognitive, substance abuse, and personality disorders.

Although there is an increase in patient demand for a more natural approach in psychiatry, only a minority of psychiatrists routinely integrate nutritional interventions into their practices. My goal is to increase the number of medical professionals who have this knowledge and can add nutrient-based psychiatry to their repertoire of treatment options.

CHAPTER 2

ADHD and Alternative Treatments

Attention-deficit/hyperactivity disorder (ADHD) is a childhood neuropsychiatric syndrome that often persists into adulthood. It is characterized by the hallmark symptoms of *inattention* (difficulty or inability to pay attention), *hyperactivity* (abnormally elevated levels of physical activity), and *impulsivity* (acting without forethought or consideration of consequences). Several subtypes exist, depending on the presenting symptoms. ADHD affects approximately 6% to 7% of children,[1] and 30% to 50% of them will also show significant symptoms as adults.[2]

The current understanding is that there is no single cause of ADHD. It does have high heritability, but that does not rule out contributions from environmental factors or genetic and environmental interactions. Conventional ADHD treatments may not be right for every person or may not be sufficient to address every symptom in various clients. The nutrient-based approach to psychiatry is an organized, systematic, and evidence-based way to complement the biochemical approaches used in psychiatry today.

Psychiatric Disorders and Nutritional Deficiencies

Some psychiatric disorders are known to be associated with specific nutritional deficiencies. Clinical depression, for example, has been associated with a number of nutritional factors, including deficiencies of protein, omega-3 fats, B vitamins, and several minerals.[3,4] Similarly, some specific nutritional deficiencies have been associated with ADHD: These include zinc, magnesium, iron, and essential fatty acids.

When these nutrients are deficient in patients with ADHD, supplementing them often improves the symptoms. Addressing known nutritional deficiencies is a well-defined type of intervention. However, the interactions among the complexities of human metabolism, dietary factors, and our limited (but growing) knowledge of genetic differences has increased our awareness that there may be patients with poorly defined nutritional deficiencies. In the case of ADHD and some other psychiatric conditions, laboratory studies are necessary to determine if there are nutrients that are suboptimal. Nutritional interventions fall into two major categories: dietary modifications and supplements.

Dietary Modifications

*Dietary modification*s are changes made to a person's diet to effect better health. They may aim to eliminate potential allergens (such as gluten, dairy, eggs, soy, etc.), chemicals (such as pesticides, contaminants, artificial food colorings and flavors, and preservatives), or excessive amounts of certain nutrient-poor substances (such as sugars, omega-6 fats, trans fats, etc.). A dietary modification can also be designed to *increase* the intake of certain foods containing beneficial nutrients, such as omega-3 fats, vitamins, minerals, antioxidants, and probiotics.

Dietary Supplements

Dietary supplements are products taken orally that contain one or more ingredients, such as vitamins or amino acids, that are intended to supplement one's diet and are *not* considered food. They may be classified as essential, metabolic, and herbal nutrients.

Essential Nutrients

Essential nutrients are given this name because they are necessary for life. Essential nutrients are composed of vitamins, minerals, and macronutrients (certain amino acids and fats) the body needs to function. The body is unable to produce these nutrients itself, so they must be supplied in the diet or by supplementation.

Metabolic Nutrients
Metabolic nutrients are substances made by the body during normal metabolism. These nutrients are long-standing elements of our evolutionary metabolisms. In the absence of medical disorders, metabolic nutrients do not need to be consumed as part of the diet because they are made in sufficient quantities by the body. They are still, however, essential for life, and if they are out of balance, the body may experience adverse reactions and ill health.

Herbal Nutrients
Herbal nutrients are plants that have medication-like effects. Certain herbs, plants, fungi, and algae are really naturally occurring drugs that sometimes also supply essential nutrients. They are neither required for life nor made by our bodies. Many herbal nutrients have healing properties as well as poisonous properties, depending on the doses and health conditions of the person taking them.

Prescription Medications
As discussed in the previous chapter, many psychiatric disorders are treated with a variety of prescription medications. The three main categories of prescription medications are as follows: fully synthetic (or manufactured), semisynthetic, and natural. Most prescription medications used in psychiatry are synthetic, but that may be changing as more research is done on the effectiveness and safety of prescribing natural interventions.

- *Synthetic medications* are chemicals that do not occur in nature and are not derived from naturally occurring substances. Synthetic medications are entirely novel chemicals. Examples include methylphenidate, fluoxetine, and clonazepam.

- *Semisynthetic medications* are derived from other naturally occurring compounds. The natural substance is modified in the laboratory to create a new manufactured medication. Examples include certain pain medications and antibiotics.

- *Natural medications* are prescription versions of naturally occurring substances that may have powerful pharmaceutical effects and should be administered only under medical supervision. Examples include prescription-strength versions of vitamins and minerals, as well as other natural substances, such as bioidentical hormones, including steroids, thyroid medications, etc.

Using Synthetic and Semisynthetic Medications

Synthetic and semisynthetic prescription medications are newly created molecules that have been in existence for only a short time and have never been part of human metabolism. It is difficult to know how such chemicals will interact with a given patient's complex biological systems, both immediately and over time. Although these unknowns pose significant potential risk, the stringent governmental regulations required to bring prescription medications to market help to lessen that risk: Large amounts of data on safety and *efficacy* (the power to produce a desired result) are systematically gathered before new medications are available to the public.

Additionally and by law, prescription medications must be administered and monitored by physicians. When appropriate, beginning with physician-prescribed, essential, and metabolic supplements with additional safety and efficacy certifications may offer the best of both intervention types, while also minimizing risk.

Using Natural Medications (Supplements and Dietary Modifications)

In contrast to prescription medications, *natural medications* (*supplements and dietary interventions*) may intervene by correcting any underlying nutritional deficiencies and optimizing various aspects of metabolism. Nutrient-based psychiatry (NBP) focuses on these types of natural interventions, which may also improve other functions important to bodily and mental health, such as synthesizing neurotransmitters. *Neurotransmitters* are chemicals that are ingested in the diet or generated by the brain that communicate information throughout the body to regulate its functions, such as movement, digestion, and breathing. Neurotransmitters affect mood, sleep, and cognition; they can also cause unfavorable symptoms when they are out of balance. Supplements and dietary modifications can address other issues important to mental and physical health, such as minimizing oxidative stress and inflammation in the body, which are discussed in greater detail in later chapters.

Nutritional Versus Prescription Approaches

In psychiatry, nutritional and prescription approaches share many of the same mechanisms of action. The term *mechanism of action* (MOA) simply refers to how a medication causes a reduction in symptoms. Both approaches have their benefits and potential negatives. Every person has a different body chemistry, unique genetic characteristics and lives in a distinct environment; how a given condition manifests and might be successfully treated differs, as well. In general, pharmaceuticals tend to be more effective at reducing symptoms than naturally occurring substances are. Therefore, they can provide rapid relief of otherwise disabling and dangerous psychiatric symptoms. However, clients may wish to avoid or minimize the use of synthetic psychotropic medications for various reasons.

Metabolic Considerations of Medications and Supplements

Because of genetic differences, age, and environmental factors, some people's metabolisms do not function optimally, which may manifest as symptoms and medical conditions that can be treated with medications and/or supplements. Before taking any medications and/or supplements, weigh the potential risks and benefits and consult with your physician. When either is taken, it creates changes in metabolism that can be neutral, beneficial, or detrimental—perhaps all three.

Importance of Education

This book, *Nutrient-Based Psychiatry,* is meant to further the dialogue between nutritional and mainstream psychiatric approaches to treating mental illnesses—reflecting the most up-to-date evidence in scientific literature, research, and clinical experience. It is *not* intended to be a final statement about how to integrate nutritional interventions into standard medical practice, but rather a way to help patients convey their desires for a more thoughtful psychiatric approach—in a format doctors can easily understand and implement.

The number of clients specifically interested in having their doctors take a natural approach in their psychiatric treatment and avoid the use of prescription medications, if possible, is growing. This is especially true in pediatric psychiatry. Data about the long-term risks of prescription medications in the developing nervous systems of children are increasing, yet there are many unknowns. Mental health consumers (especially parents) often take more time to educate themselves in this regard, although much partial information and misinformation on the subject of nutritional and prescription interventions still exists. The more research a client (or client's parents) can do about the different treatment options for ADHD, the better they will feel about their course of action.

PART TWO: THE SCIENCE BEHIND NUTRIENT-BASED PSYCHIATRY®

Part Two of the text is primarily written for medical professionals; however, some adult patients and parents of children with ADHD may find the science behind nutrient-based psychiatry informative and interesting. Again, this book is *not* intended to be a do-it-yourself guide. Rather, its purpose is to convey how the principles of NBP may be useful in ADHD management and encourage interested readers to give the information designed for physicians to their medical practitioners.

Chapter 3

Rationale for Using Nutritional Supplements and Dietary Interventions in Psychiatry: It's Complicated

Sometimes it's best to start at the beginning to understand a complicated topic, especially one that encompasses the brain. Our bodies are composed of matter. Atoms are considered the primary functional units of matter; they are microscopic particles composed of variable numbers of protons, neutrons, and electrons. Protons and neutrons form the nucleus of the atom, and the electrons orbit it, much like planets orbit the sun.

Atoms appear to be almost entirely empty space and are held together by electromagnetic forces. They combine to form simple and quite complex arrangements known as *molecules*, which are not yet living material. For example, water is a simple molecule composed of two hydrogen atoms and one oxygen atom. Deoxyribonucleic acid (DNA) is a highly complex molecule that encodes the genetic instructions used in the development and functioning of all known living organisms.

Cell Structure
Molecules, in turn, make up organelles, cytoplasm (the fluid inside of our cells), and membranes that constitute the various cells of our bodies. With some exceptions, the cell is the simplest unit of matter that is alive; cells are made up of millions of molecules. A single cell can be a living organism (such as yeast or bacterium) or a part of larger organisms. Groups of similar types of cells make up the different tissues of our bodies, such as muscle tissue, connective tissue, and nervous tissue. Similar types of tissue form organs, such as the brain, heart, and skin. Organs working together to perform a specific function are part an organ system. For example, the brain, spinal cord, and peripheral nerves constitute the body's nervous system.

Finally, a group of organ systems makes up an *organism*, or an individual living thing, such as a human, fish, or lizard.

Neurotransmitters and the Human Brain

The brain is composed of billions of cells called *neurons*, each connected to other neurons via pathways called *synapses*. These connections allow neurons to communicate with each other using neurotransmitters (NTs) as the messengers. NTs are substances made by neurons, ingested in the diet or taken as a dietary supplement. Some of the most common NTs in the human brain are acetylcholine (Ach), serotonin (5-hydroxytryptamine), dopamine (DA), norepinephrine (NE), and gamma-aminobutyric acid (GABA), just to name a few. In simple terms, when a neuron wants to send a message, it releases NTs into the synapse, which attach to receptor sites (RSs). *Receptor sites* are proteins folded into particular shapes that are embedded within the neuron membrane. See Figure 1 in the following chapter.

When bound to an RS, NTs effect changes in the receiving neuron's *metabolism*, or life-sustaining chemical transformations within cells. Each NT can bind to a number of different receptor subtypes. For example, dopamine can bind to receptors sites D1–D5. The brain has the ability to adapt to changes in the environment and behavior by constantly reinforcing and rearranging its structure. This ability is known as *neuroplasticity*.

DNA contains our genetic material or genes. Genes are sections of DNA that store the blueprints for making proteins out of chains of amino acids strung together in specific sequences. These proteins serve as enzymes, RSs, messengers to turn off and on other genes, and structural components of our bodies. *Enzymes* are complex proteins that allow necessary chemical reactions to take place. Proteins also fold into intricate shapes to form receptor sites and other structures that automatically carry out the business of our cells: taking in nutrients, eliminating waste, producing energy, making repairs, reacting to the environment, etc. The sum total of all of these tasks and reactions is our body's metabolism.

Psychotropic Medications in Psychiatry

In general, pharmaceuticals are more effective at creating changes in biochemistry than naturally occurring substances are. Therefore, they can provide rapid relief from otherwise incapacitating and dangerous psychiatric symptoms and are one type of biochemical intervention. The vast majority of psychotropic medications prescribed in psychiatry target the release and metabolism of NTs or interact directly with receptor sites. These actions then alter the metabolism of neurons and, over time, can change the brain's structure and its connections via neuroplasticity.

For example, in the case of depression, increased levels of the NT serotonin may alleviate symptoms; the class of medications known as *selective serotonin reuptake inhibitors* (SSRIs) tends to do this reliably and safely. I'm not aware of any naturally occurring supplements with this type of robust and highly specific effect on serotonin. Unfortunately, there are also cases in which increased levels of serotonin do not seem to help significantly. Interventions with other mechanisms of action (MOAs) are necessary when the conventional medication approach isn't working. Although these can include psychotherapy and behavioral interventions, other biochemical approaches used in NBP may also successfully treat the condition.

Chapter 4

Dietary Supplements as a Nutritional Intervention

Dietary supplements are often prescribed to address nutritional deficiencies and optimize certain aspects of metabolism. They are considered another form of treatment for a number of illnesses; in this book, their abilities to effect positive change in ADHD patients is explored. Supplements can come in the form of pills, capsules, powders, or drinks.

Categories and Characteristics of Dietary Supplements

The Food and Drug Administration (FDA) defines a dietary supplement as an ingested product that contains a "dietary ingredient" intended to add further nutritional value to supplement the diet.[5] The following are examples of dietary ingredients used in NBP.

Essential Nutrients

Essential nutrients are given this name because they are necessary for life, and the body is unable to produce them. Therefore, they must be supplied in the diet or by supplementation. These nutrients are long-standing elements of our evolutionary metabolisms and include vitamins, minerals, essential fatty acids, amino acids, and probiotics.

Vitamins are organic compounds essential for the normal functioning of metabolism and must be obtained from dietary sources. Vitamins may act as enzyme cofactors in metabolic reactions, have hormone-like activity, and/or function as antioxidants (such as vitamin C).

Dietary minerals are chemical elements required for life and must be obtained from the diet. Minerals serve as electrolytes and cofactors for enzymatic metabolic reactions; they also have structural roles in the human body. For example, calcium helps to form the skeletal system.

Essential fatty acids (EFAs) are fats required for life, cannot be synthesized by the body, and must be obtained from dietary sources. They include the omega-3 and omega-6 fatty acids. In part, EFAs determine the structure and function of cellular membranes, which affect metabolism and communications between cells. EFAs also influence genetic expression; bodily inflammation; and the *endocannabinoid* system, a group of lipids (fats) and their receptors involved in appetite, pain sensation, memory, mood, and behavior. Refer to Figure 1.

Probiotics are microorganisms thought to be beneficial to the host organism. There are an estimated 500 to 1,000 species of bacteria living in the human gastrointestinal tract. In the body, bacterial cells outnumber human cells by at least 10 to one. Intestinal microorganisms are a virtual inner organ, with a large volume of genetic material that is actually greater than that of our own DNA.[6] They may be found in fermented foods like yogurt and in the soil and may be taken as dietary supplements.

Metabolic Nutrients
Metabolic nutrients, conversely, are made by the body but are still essential for life. These include such metabolic inter-mediates as amino acid derivatives and phospholipids.

Amino acids and their derivatives are building blocks of proteins that form enzymes and body tissues. Some amino acids, including lysine, phenylalanine, and tryptophan, are essential (meaning they must be obtained from dietary sources) or are essential under certain metabolic conditions. They may act as neurotransmitters or are the precursors to neurotransmitters.

Phospholipids, such as phosphatidylserine (PS) and phospha-tidylcholine (PC) are major components of cell membranes that help to form the *phospholipid bilayer,* which is a thin membrane made up of two layers of lipid (fat) molecules that form a continuous barrier around cells.[7] Phospholipids are synthesized inside the cells, and small amounts are obtained from dietary sources. They have many functions in cellular structure and metabolism. To a large extent, the types of lipids in the membrane determine its physical characteristics and the functioning of transmembrane proteins and receptor sites embedded within it. The term *membrane-lipid therapy* refers to treatments (medications and supplements) that target membrane structure and function. See Figure 1.

Figure 1: Fluid Mosaic Model of the Cellular Membrane

Extracellular space

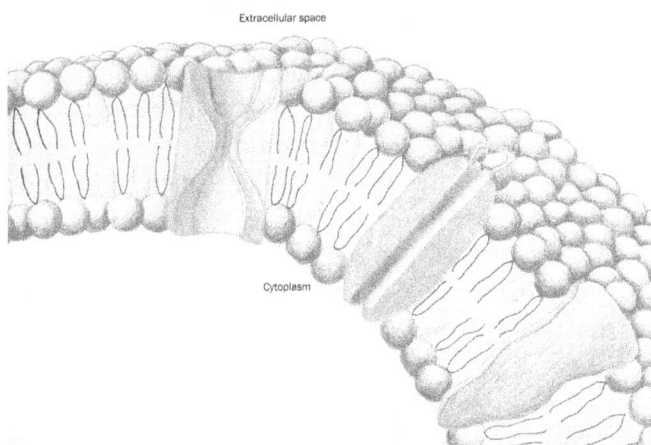

Cytoplasm

Phospholipids and essential fatty acids in the body tend to accumulate here.

Herbal Nutrients
Certain herbs, plants, fungi, and algae are actually naturally occurring drugs that sometimes also supply essential nutrients. Examples include chamomile, ginkgo biloba, and green tea. They are not required for life and are not made by our bodies. *Medicinal herbs* are plants that contain *phytochemicals* (or chemicals found in plants that have biological significance), which have various medication-like effects on

the human body. Many herbs have cultural medicinal uses dating back thousands of years.

Generally Recognized as Safe (GRAS)

The essential and metabolic nutritional supplements tend to have Generally Recognized as Safe (GRAS) status granted by the FDA, prescription versions, and uses recognized by mainstream medicine. See Table 1. Although medicinal herbs often have long histories of human consumption, and evidence and use for medicinal purposes is increasing, they often do not have GRAS status. In general, medicinal herbs may be thought of as combination formulas, often having multiple active constituents—each with potential affinities for multiple metabolic targets.

This leads to a wide range of additive and/or contradicting effects, some of which may be desired and therapeutic, while others may be unnecessary and produce adverse effects. It is often unclear which active herbal ingredients are good for specific indications. Herbs are commonly standardized to a certain percentage of (what is presumed to be) the active constituent, but that may not take into account the medicinal properties of other components.

Relatively less is known about the *pharmacodynamics* (physiological effects of chemicals on organisms, the mechanisms of action, and the relationship between chemical concentration and effect), safety, toxicity, and long-term use of herbs as compared to essential and metabolic supplements. Although there is some compelling evidence that certain herbs may be useful in addressing psychiatric and medical conditions, many have hormonal and endocrine effects that could potentially make them harmful in certain populations, including children and adolescents.

Table 1: Characteristics of Three Types of Dietary Supplements Versus Synthetic Medications

	Essential Supplements	Metabolic Supplements	Herbal Supplements	Synthetic and Semisynthetic Medication
Necessary for life?	Yes	Yes	No	No
Made by the body?	No	Yes	No	No
Naturally occurring?	Yes	Yes	Yes	No
Prescription forms?	Often	Sometimes	Uncommon	Yes
GRAS?*	Almost always	Often	Sometimes	n/a
Long history of medicinal use in man?	No	No	Often	No

*Generally recognized as safe (GRAS) is a status granted by the FDA, indicating that a substance added to food is considered safe under conditions of intended use, as assessed by a consensus of experts.

Current Good Manufacturing Practice (CGMP)

The current good manufacturing practice (CGMP) regulations are enforced by the US FDA and provide systems that monitor and control drug and supplement manufacturing processes and facilities. Such factors as content, strength, quality, and purity are closely monitored.[8] Certain companies that manufacture dietary supplements can apply for and obtain a good manufacturing practice (GMP) certification from the GMP Certification Organization, which is a nonprofit entity that inspects and certifies that the facility where the supplement is manufactured meets the appropriate standards. GMP certification is awarded on an annual basis.[9] Another entity that registers and monitors facilities where nutritional supplements are manufactured is the division of the NSF International for dietary supplement certification. This certification, which includes a GMP facility inspection, has standards developed with input from the FDA; National Institutes of Health; and other governmental, industry, and consumer groups and ensures that supplements do not contain unacceptable levels of contaminants.[10] Prescribing and choosing dietary supplements manufactured by companies that have these certifications helps to ensure that the product reflects label information.

Prescribing Supplements and Medications

The difference in regulations for supplements versus medications contributes to prescribing considerations. Prescription medications are regulated for safety, efficacy, and purity by the FDA prior to being made available for public consumption. Once on the market, prescription medications are continually monitored for safety in a systematic way.

Manufacturers of dietary supplements, however, are not required to prove to the FDA that their products are safe or effective—as long as they don't claim to prevent, treat, or cure any specific disease. The FDA steps in only when safety issues arise.[11] Additionally, supplements may not actually contain the amount of the active ingredient(s) claimed on the label and/or may include other potentially *toxic substances* (contaminants). The actual amounts of ingredients can vary between brands or even among different batches of the same brand. This fact is a major drawback of prescribing supplements medicinally.

However, it is often the case that supplements are recognized as having evidence-based medicinal uses as reflected by prescription versions and qualified health claims. A *qualified health claim*[12] is an FDA-approved claim, supported by credible scientific evidence, regarding a relationship between a substance and a health-related condition. Moreover, supplements with GRAS status have evidence of safety when used as intended. This type of additional safety and efficacy information associated with many supplements improves physicians' confidence when prescribing them.

A possible advantage to using a naturally occurring nutrient is that as part of our long-standing evolutionary metabolism, our bodies are familiar with its structure and function. However, when supplements without GRAS status are used, the risks include contamination, adverse events, and lack of efficacy. Using supplements that have been on the market for a long time, have prescription versions, have qualified health claims, have GRAS status, are manufactured under the dietary supplement CGMP guidelines, and are administered by an experienced health care professional helps to minimize those risks.

It may be difficult to anticipate how prescription medications will interact with complex biological systems in the short term and over time. When clinically appropriate, starting off with physician-prescribed, essential, and metabolic supplements that have additional safety and efficacy certifications may provide the best of both intervention types. Although the goal is to obtain symptom relief while minimizing risk, this type of approach largely lies in uncharted territory. Therefore, potential interactions between nutritional interventions and medications require professional surveillance.

Chapter 5

How Pharmaceutical and Nutritional Interventions Work

Nutritional interventions that address psychiatric conditions use the same proposed mechanisms of action as prescription medications, along with several unique mechanisms of action (MOAs). Behavior, cognition, and emotion are largely influenced by neurotransmitters interacting with membrane-associated proteins located on and within the phospholipid bilayer (membrane) of neurons. When activated, the proteins set off cascades of events that affect neuron function and communication.

Prescription psychiatric medications are believed to work by influencing neurotransmitter release and/or deactivation or by interacting directly with receptor sites. For example, selective serotonin reuptake inhibitors (SSRIs), which are frequently used in psychiatry, inhibit the deactivation of the neurotransmitter serotonin by preventing it from being taken back up into the presynaptic neuron. Acetylcholinesterase is the enzyme that breaks down the neurotransmitter acetylcholine (Ach). Medications that inhibit this enzyme lead to increased levels of Ach, which is therapeutic in the treatment of Alzheimer's disease. Bupropion, a widely used prescription antidepressant, not only inhibits the reuptake of dopamine (DA) and norepinephrine (NE) but also stimulates their release. Benzodiazepine medications, which are used for anxiety, interact directly with the receptor site complex for the neurotransmitter gamma-aminobutyric acid (GABA).

These mechanisms of action can also be the main effects of interventions used in NBP. This is especially true of metabolic and herbal supplements. In contrast to prescription medications, supplements may intervene by correcting any underlying nutritional deficiencies, improving the synthesis of neurotransmitters, minimizing oxidative stress and inflammation, optimizing the functions of the immune system, and modifying the structure and functioning of neuronal membranes (phospholipid bilayer).

Nutritional Deficiencies

Nutritional deficiencies may arise in several different ways. Although malnutrition commonly results in nutritional deficiencies, the shortcomings of industrialized food production, along with peer- and media-influenced eating patterns, can lead to nutritional deficiencies in the face of adequate or often excess caloric intake.

A study of food intakes in the US population from 2001 and 2002 published in the *Journal of the American Dietetic Association* concluded that instead of consuming foods that are nutrient dense, Americans tend to consume foods high in fats and added sugars.[13] Foods such as sweetened soft drinks, grain-based desserts, nonskim dairy products, and fatty meats do *not* contain the recommended nutritional intake. Another study on food sources of energy and nutrients among US adults from 2003 to 2006 concluded that a large proportion of total energy comes from energy-dense, low-nutrient foods.[14] The main culprits were cakes, cookies, pies, and soft drinks.

These poor dietary choices call for effective strategies to improve diet quality with healthier, nutrient-dense foods and reduce caloric consumption by US adults.[15] A 1997 study on children's and adolescents' food intakes in the United States as compared with the recommended daily allowances found that only approximately 30% met the recommended intakes for fruits, grains, meat, and dairy, and only 36% met the recommended intake for vegetables.[16] Shockingly, only 1% met all of the daily nutritional intake recommendations, and 16% met none of them. The authors concluded that interventions are needed.

Antinutrients

Antinutrients are synthetic and naturally occurring compounds that adversely affect the absorption of nutrients.[17] Common sources of these substances are prescription and over-the-counter (OTC) medications and various foods. Examples of antinutrients found in foods include phytic acid (may decrease absorption of phosphorus, calcium, copper, iron, magnesium and zinc), tannins (may decrease absorption of iron and zinc), oxalates (may decrease absorption of calcium and magnesium), fiber in excessive amounts (may decrease absorption of calcium, iron , zinc and magnesium) and glucosino-lates (may decrease absorption of iodine). Additionally, a number of antinutrients may interfere with the action of digestive enzymes potentially impairing the absorption of many nutrients. Fermenta-tion and cooking can decrease the amounts of antinutrients in foods like grains and legumes.[18] Food choices that are low in nutrients and high in calories, genetically influenced metabolic differences and the ingestion of antinutrients can increase the need for essen-tial nutrients. Refer to Table 2 for examples. Consuming the recom-mended daily allowance of vitamins, minerals, and macronutrients (fats, proteins, and carbohydrates) may not necessarily prevent nutritional deficiencies.

Psychiatric Disorders and Nutritional Deficiencies

Some psychiatric disorders are known to correlate with specific nutritional deficiencies. Clinical depression, for example, has been associated with a number of nutritional factors, including deficien-cies of protein, omega-3 fats, B vitamins, and several minerals.[19,20]

Table 2: Examples of Commonly Prescribed Medications That Can Adversely Affect Nutrient Availability

Nutrient Affected	Medication/Food Component
Intestinal flora (probiotics)	Antibiotics
Folic acid	Anti-convulsants, anti-diabetics, anti-ulcer medications, diuretics, NSAIDS, aspirin, serotonin specific reuptake inhibitors (SSRI), birth control pills
Vitamin B6	Antibiotics, diuretics, BCP, estrogens
Vitamin B12	Anti-convulsants, BCP, anti-ulcer medications, anti-diabetics
Magnesium	Antibiotics, corticosteroids, diuretics, BCP, estrogens, antacids
Zinc	Ace inhibitors, diuretics, anti-ulcer medications, corticosteroids, BCP, estrogens
Coenzyme Q10 (CoQ10):	Statin medications, beta blockers, clonidine, anti-diabetics

These are examples of commonly prescribed medications that can adversely affect nutrient availability. Correcting for these interactions via supplementa-tion with the affected nutrient may be necessary. Efforts can also be made to minimize or eliminate certain medications, when possible.

In considering metabolic influences in psychiatric conditions, the synthesis and deactivation of neurotransmitters is paramount. Multiple-step metabolic reactions are responsible for these processes. Each reaction requires an enzyme; many also require the presence of cofactors, which are the essential vitamins and minerals that must be obtained from the diet.[21] For example, vitamins B1, B3, and B6; folate; iron; calcium; magnesium; zinc; and vitamin C are the cofactors necessary for the synthesis of the neurotransmitter serotonin and subsequently its metabolism to *melatonin*, a hormone essential to establishing and maintaining our circadian (sleep/wake) cycles.

Similarly, multiple vitamins and minerals (including copper) are required for the synthesis of the neurotransmitters DA and NE. The complexity of these metabolic pathways is compounded by the fact that many of the B vitamins in these reactions must undergo modifications to transform them into their activated forms. The activated forms allow them to function as coenzymes, another complex process that is, in turn, dependent upon the presence of various nutrients.

Genetic Disorders

DNA is a complex molecule located inside the nucleus of our cells. It contains the information necessary to create the structure and carry out the metabolic processes of our bodies. Genes are sections of DNA that contain a code that is used to make all of the proteins our bodies are capable of making. These proteins then form the structure of our bodies (such as muscle tissue, for example), *enzymes* (proteins that allow chemical transformations to take place), and the receptor sites that lay embedded within the membranes of our cells.

Mutations are changes to our DNA over time that, depending upon the location and nature of the change, may have a significant effect on the structure or function of our bodies. Mutations typically arise from radiation or chemical *mutagens* (agents that cause mutations) and errors in replication. One important way mutations can affect our metabolism is that they can alter genes that code for enzymes. When this occurs, detrimental changes to our metabolism can result. A 2002 article in the *American Journal of Clinical Nutrition* points out that about one-third of genetic mutations lead to the corresponding enzyme having a decreased binding affinity for its coenzyme, which leads to a decreased reaction rate.[22] Put simply, genetic mutations can make certain metabolic pathways, such as the synthesis of neurotransmitters, sluggish.

There are about 50 human genetic disorders that can be treated by supplementing high doses of the vitamin cofactor for the corresponding enzyme. This results in at least a partial restoration of the enzyme's activity.[23] By supplementing the diet with the correct vitamins and minerals, even enzymes with decreased activity become supersaturated, leading to recovery of near-normal enzyme functions.[24] This raises the possibility that the recommended daily allowances of vitamins and minerals may not be the same for everyone. Genetic differences, aging, and the ingestion of antinutrients may cause the need for much higher doses of certain vitamins and minerals in some people to compensate for limited enzymatic function.

We are still in the process of discovering additional defective enzymes that would be responsive to therapeutic vitamin and mineral supplementation. When more information about genomics and mutations becomes available, it may be possible to prescribe customized nutritional therapies to suit specific individual needs. However, for now, high-dose vitamin and mineral supplementation is a reasonable, safe, and potentially therapeutic strategy.[25]

Oxidative Stress and Psychiatric Disorders

Most psychiatric disorders are associated with *oxidative stress*.[26] See Figures 2 through 4. These disorders include most mood disorders, anxiety disorders, psychotic disorders, substance abuse disorders, and developmental disorders. In the simplest terms, oxidative stress is caused by the presence of free radicals, shown on the left side of Figure 2. *Free radicals* basically attack and damage other healthy molecules present because they have an unpaired electron in their outermost shells, making them highly unstable and reactive. Antioxidants, shown on the right side of Figure 2, may be likened to a storehouse of available electrons. *Antioxidants* neutralize the effect of free radicals and prevent them from harming your body by donating an electron, creating a pair of electrons that will stabilize the free radical.

Figure 2: Oxidative Stress and Free Radicals

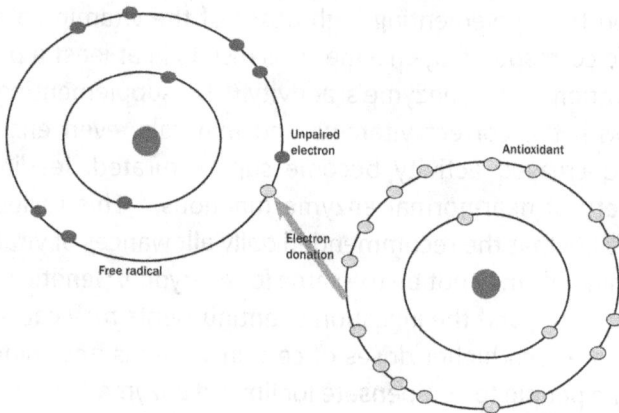

The availability of both endogenous (made by the body) and exogenous (ingested in the diet) antioxidants helps to protect our tissues from free radical damage.

Mitochondria Create Free Radicals
Structures called *mitochondria*, which specialize in creating energy (in the form of adenosine triphosphate) from glucose and oxygen, live inside cells. Scientists believe that around two billion years ago, mitochondria were bacteria living outside of higher organisms. Over time, it appears they migrated to the intracellular space of more complex organisms, finally leading to a symbiotic relationship that persists today.

Our bodies provide mitochondria with glucose and oxygen, and they make our energy. This relationship is the source of the energy that drives virtually all metabolic processes in our bodies. Mitochondria can be likened to internal combustion engines. As such, they give off exhaust in the form of free radicals, which are by-products of energy production.

If sufficient antioxidants from both endogenous (antioxidants that are made by our bodies) and exogenous (antioxidants that we consume in our diets) sources are available, then free radicals are stabilized. If, however, excessive amounts of free radicals are produced or not enough antioxidants are present to stabilize them, the excess free radicals attempt to take electrons from various tissues of our bodies, including our cellular membranes, proteins, the DNA of the mitochondria themselves, and the nuclear DNA.

Collectively, this situation contributes to cellular dysfunction, metabolic disorders, cell mutation, *carcinogenesis* (cancer formation), and the creation of more free radicals and less energy. Ideally, there is enough of a balance in the body between free radical production and antioxidants to neutralize them before significant damage occurs. Refer to Figure 3.

Figure 3: The Balance Between Free Radical Formation and Antioxidants

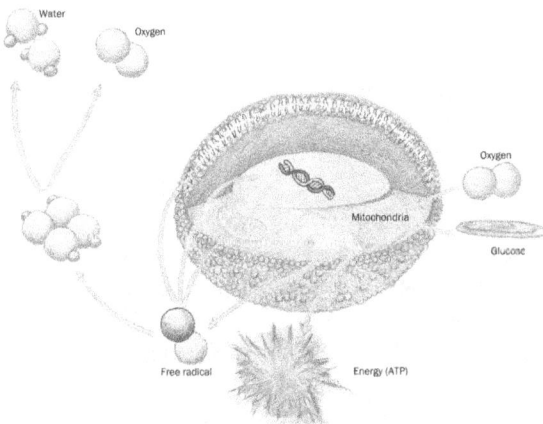

Water
Oxygen
Oxygen
Mitochondria
Glucose
Free radical
Energy (ATP)

The creation of free radicals is a natural by-product of cellular metabolism.

Additional Sources of Free Radicals

As our mitochondria and the DNA contained within them age, they tend to produce more free radicals and less energy. If we consume many more calories than necessary, we burn more glucose and oxygen, which creates more free radicals. Chronic infection; cellular inflammation; and environmental toxins, including pollutants, illicit drugs and prescription medications, ultraviolet and ionizing radiation, and physical and psychological stress are also sources of excessive free radical production that lead to cellular dysfunction.[27] See Figure 4. The fact that psychological stress is associated with oxidative stress helps to explain why most psychiatric disorders are also associated with increased oxidative stress.

Figure 4: Sources of Oxidative Stress

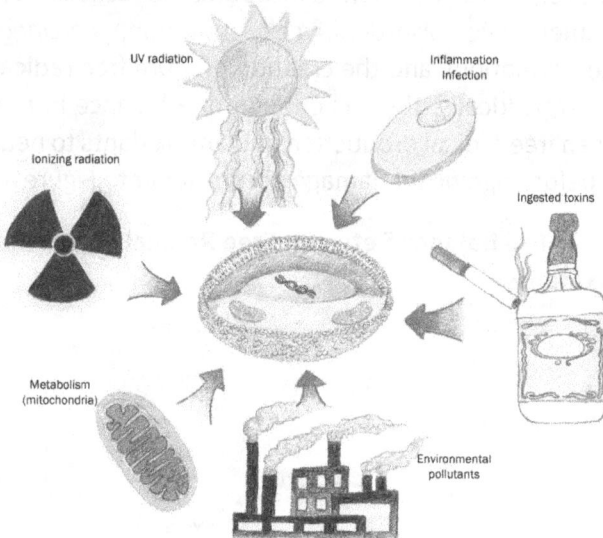

In addition to mitochondria producing free radicals during normal cellular respiration, there are many other sources.

Immuno-Inflammatory-Oxidative Axis

The immune system, inflammation, and oxidative stress (also called the *immuno-inflammatory-oxidative axis* or *IIO axis*) are highly complex and interdependent yet necessary systems.

Some psychiatric disorders are associated with inflammation (see Figure 5) and immune system dysfunction: Depression is probably the best researched in this regard.[28] Nearly all of the nutritional interventions used in NBP have antioxidant, anti-inflammatory, and/or immunomodulating properties. In order to grasp a major benefit of NBP, we must have an understanding of these systems and how they contribute to psychiatric disorders.

Inflammation and Immune System Dysfunction

The innate immune system defends against infection and repairs the tissues of our body by initiating a complex cascade of events called *inflammation*. For example, in Figure 5, the skin has been broken and bacteria are threatening infection. A type of immune cell, known as a *mast cell,* detects the situation and releases factors to dilate the local blood vessels, thereby enlarging them and increasing blood flow to the affected area. Another type of immune cell, known as a *neutrophil*, goes beyond the walls of the dilated vessels and migrates to the threatened area. The neutrophils engulf the invading bacteria in a process known as *phagocytosis*.

Figure 5: Inflammation

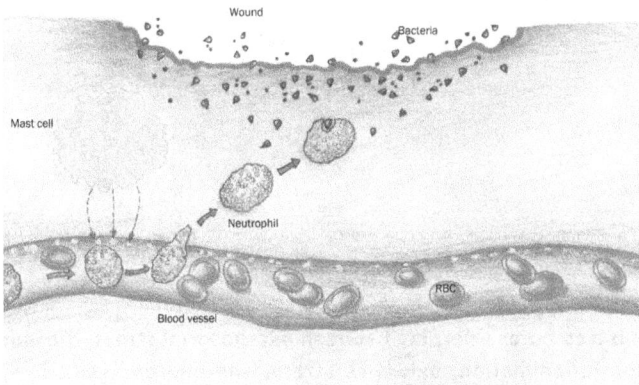

Once inside the cell, a free radical attack, also known as an *oxidative burst*, is used to kill the bacteria.

Targeted free radical attacks destroy viruses; parasites; and cancerous, precancerous, and aging cells. If inflammation is acute and limited, it can heal tissues and fight infection and tumor growth. However, chronic or long-term inflammation is a critical factor contributing to a vast number of medical disorders. These include neurologic and psychiatric disorders; metabolic disorders; multiple types of cancer; bone, muscular, and skeletal disorders; and cardiovascular diseases.

Psychosocial Stressors and the Immune System

Chronic inflammation can arise from the aging process, infection, dietary choices, obesity, lack of exercise and sleep, chronic exposure to allergens, genetic factors, and psychosocial stressors. The term *psychosocial stressors* refers to stress originating from interactions with people and/or the environment, including things like natural disasters, financial and economic concerns, interpersonal conflicts, illnesses, and death of friends and family. See Figure 6. Once again, we gain an insight into why many psychiatric disorders are associated with inflammation and immune system dysfunction.

Figure 6: The Psychosocial Stressor Feedback Loop

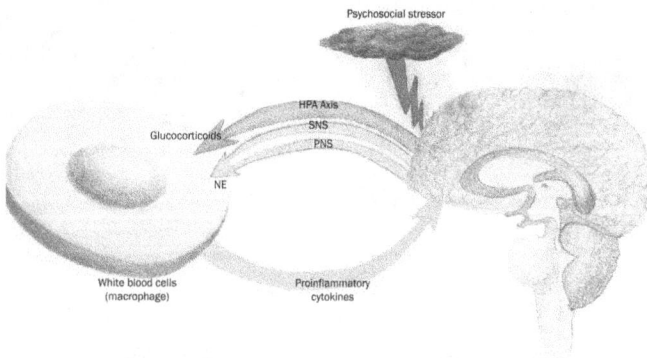

Psychosocial stressor

HPA Axis
SNS
PNS

Glucocorticoids

NE

White blood cells
(macrophage)

Proinflammatory
cytokines

There is a complex interplay between psychosocial stress, the immune system, inflammation, oxidative stress, and neuropsychiatric symptoms.

In Figure 6, the psychosocial stressor (represented by the light-ening bolt), which may be an actual or perceived threat, deacti-vates the *parasympathetic nervous system (PNS)*, the branch of the autonomic nervous system that is active when the body is at rest or relaxed. The stressor activates the *hypothalamic pitu-itary adrenal (HPA) axis*, a major part of the neuroendocrine system that controls the body's reaction to stress and regu-lates such processes as digestion and the immune system, and the *sympathetic nervous system (SNS)*, a branch of the autonomic nervous system that regulates the body's reaction to stress by activating the fight-or-flight response. This leads to the release of norepinephrine and glucocorticoids, such as cortisol, that affect cells in the immune system, including *macrophages,* a specialized type of white blood cell. This, in turn, may lead to immunosuppression with an increased risk of infection, as well as immunoactivation with the associated release of proinflammatory cytokines.

Cortisol and proinflammatory cytokines gain access to the central nervous system, creating increased oxidative stress and influencing virtually every aspect of brain function—including neurotransmitter metabolism; neuroendocrine func-tion; synaptic plasticity; and neurocircuits that regulate mood, motor activity, and motivation, potentially leading to symp-toms that are associated with various psychiatric disorders, such as depression, fatigue, lack of appetite, an inability to think clearly, and the inability to initiate and maintain sleep or excessive sleep (*hypersomnia*).[29]

Various treatments used in psychology, psychiatry, and medi-cine intervene at different stages of the complex process of reducing psychosocial stressors. Psychotherapies may be effec-tive in lessening the client's perception of the stressor and help the person feel safe and supported while gaining insight into the nature and origin of the symptoms that are troubling him or her. Social interventions may remove a client from dangerous and stressful situations. Interventions that activate the relaxation response (*parasympathetic nervous system*), such as exercise, yoga, diaphragmatic breathing, and meditation, as well as certain NBP interventions and medications, may decrease over-activation of the HPA axis and sympathetic nervous system.

We can also employ cortisol-lowering, immunomodulating, anti-inflammatory, and/or antioxidant NBP dietary and supplement interventions. These will decrease the influx of proinflammatory cytokines, glucocorticoids, and immune cells into the central nervous system (CNS). Finally, psychiatric interventions may employ medications and NBP approaches that address the situation at the neurotransmitter and receptor site levels, such as SSRIs.

Treating psychiatric disorders is not a one-size-fits-all proposition. It is important to meet the patient where he or she is. Certain clients are more amenable to and accepting of specific approaches. Be flexible and offer many different potentially effective interventions to arrive at the specific combination that works for each client.

In addition to expected actions on neurotransmitters and at receptor sites, virtually all nutritional interventions used in NBP regulate the immuno-inflammatory-oxidative axis (IIO axis). Balance in this regard is essential, as some level of oxidative stress and free radicals is necessary for life as part of our normal metabolism—to fight off infection and stop the proliferation of cancerous and precancerous cells. Adequate amounts of antioxidants prevent free radicals from damaging our tissues, including DNA, fats, and proteins.

The immune system regulates inflammation, which is also necessary to fight infection and tumor growth. Immunosuppression, which can arise from chronic stress, tends to increase the risk of infection. Conversely, overactivation of the immune system and inflammation associated with autoimmune disorders and allergic reactions lead to chronic inflammation and a host of other disorders. The ability of nutritional interventions to regulate the IIO axis may be partly, or in some cases solely, responsible for their therapeutic effects, may address or prevent comorbidities associated with some psychiatric disorders, and may benefit the overall health of clients. These are prime reasons NBP should be considered at some point during treatment.

Membranes, Fats, and Neurological Function

The phospholipid bilayer that makes up the membranes of our neurons is composed of a vast array of *lipids* (fats). Lipids form transient and stable structures, serving as the platforms for the activity and interactions of proteins that constitute cellular communication.[30] Refer back to Figure 1. This membrane represents an important therapeutic target for a number of medical and psychiatric disorders.

Membrane lipids are involved in crucial cell functions. The lipid structure of the membrane governs the activities of membrane-associated enzymes, receptor sites, and transporters, which, in turn, influence various cascades of events that determine cellular functions, including cell signaling and genetic expression. Oxidation of membrane fats (known as *lipid peroxidation*) results in changes to shapes and physical properties of the membranes. The process of lipid peroxidation is a result of oxidative stress that is composed of a set of chain reactions culminating in cellular damage due to increased water permeability, membrane rigidity, calcium influx, and cell death.[31]

Such damage can also alter the function of serotonin and dopamine transporters located within the membranes.[32] Products that evolve from lipid peroxidation cause further damage to cellular structures, DNA, and enzymes.[33] Elevated lipid peroxidation is a well-established feature common to nearly all psychiatric conditions, including depression,[34] bipolar,[35] psychotic,[36] anxiety,[37] substance abuse,[38] sleep,[39] and developmental disorders.[40] In many cases, the degree of lipid peroxidation directly correlates with symptom severity.

Membrane-Lipid Therapies

Specific lipid therapies, both naturally occurring and synthetic, may be developed to treat a variety of diseases, such as cancer; hypertension; obesity; and neurodegenerative, metabolic, and autoimmune conditions; Escribá uses the term *membrane-lipid therapy* to describe the class of interventions that target the structure and functioning of cellular membranes, which contrasts with conventional therapies that commonly target proteins, including receptor sites and intracellular proteins.[41] Both forms of therapy, however, aim to regulate protein activity.

Antioxidant Interventions

A number of antioxidant interventions that specifically address damage to membrane lipids by preventing lipid peroxidation may also be considered a form of membrane-lipid therapy. NBP uses a membrane therapy approach in two ways: Antioxidant interventions prevent lipid peroxidation, thereby preserving membrane integrity, and essential fatty acids and phospholipids are supplemented directly to ensure an adequate supply. The latter approach includes dietary interventions, as well as supplementing with omega-3 fats and phosphatidylserine, in the case of ADHD and other psychiatric conditions. By addressing underlying alterations in the types and/or levels of membrane lipids, antioxidant and lipid interventions can profoundly influence neurotransmitter-receptor site interactions and intracellular events down to the genetic level.

In Table 3, note that prescription psychiatric medications are *not* known to address neurotransmitter synthesis or membrane-lipid dysfunction, but some have been shown to address aspects of oxidative stress and inflammation. These actions may be responsible for a portion of the clinically observed therapeutic effects. Essential and certain metabolic nutrients are unique in their abilities to influence neurotransmitter synthesis. Essential fatty acids and phospholipids are unique in their ability to regulate membrane-lipid content and subsequent cellular activities. Some antioxidants that prevent lipid peroxidation affect the quality and state of membrane lipids.

Table 3: Comparison of Mechanisms of Action (MOAs) Addressed by Various Types of Biochemical Interventions Used in Psychiatry and NBP

	NT Synthesis	NT Release	NT Deactivation	Direct RS Interaction	IIO Axis	Membrane Lipid Therapy
Prescription Psychiatric Medications	No	Yes	Yes	Yes	Yes: SSRI	No
Essential Nutrients	Yes: AA, vitamins, minerals	No	No	Yes: AA, vitamins, minerals	Yes	Yes: EFA
Metabolic Supplements	Yes: AA derivatives	Yes	No	Yes: AA derivatives	Yes	Yes: phospholipids
Herbs	No	Yes	Yes	Yes	Yes	Possibly

Comparison of MOAs addressed by various types of biochemical interventions used in psychiatry and NBP: NT = neurotransmitter; RS = receptor site; IIO = immuno-inflammatory-oxidative; SSRI = selective serotonin reuptake inhibitor; AA = amino acid; EFA = essential fatty acid.

Chapter 6

How Nutrient-Based Psychiatry®
(NBP) Works

Developing a nutrient-based approach for a particular psychiatric condition requires a critical evaluation of the safety and efficacy evidence of specific nutritional interventions. Those with a favorable risk-to-benefit ratio can then be implemented, in essentially the same way as prescription medications. Ideally, the evidence base for the efficacy of a medical intervention comes from well-designed, randomized controlled trials published in peer-reviewed journals. When compared with the evidence for prescription medications, the strength of the evidence for the efficacy of nutritional interventions is limited by the number and quality of trials. Additionally, more safety and efficacy data are systemically collected for prescription medications.

To a significant degree, the evidence base for a medication or supplement follows the research funding. For the most part, nutrient-based approaches are not patentable, and exclusive manufacturing and distribution rights are not granted to any one company. Therefore, limited evidence for the efficacy of a naturally occurring treatment may actually be indicating limited profitability.

Over the last few decades, and particularly over the last few years, there has been an increase in the volume of information in the medical literature about the efficacy and safety of nutrient-based approaches in psychiatry and medicine. When a threshold is reached, it becomes possible to develop evidence-based treatment strategies for the management of psychiatric conditions.

NBP Protocol
The NBP protocol is based on using nutritional interventions

in a systematic and categorical way. Depending on presentation as well as the desires of the client, NBP may be integrated with prescription medications or used in lieu of them. When prescription medications are necessary, they may be used in conjunction with NBP approaches at any time, while taking into account potential medication-nutrient interactions. Certain types of clinical situations, such as clients in an inpatient setting and the presence of dangerous or incapacitating symptoms, require immediate intervention with prescription psychotropics. In such cases, it may be more appropriate to consider nutritional factors *after* a degree of stability and symptom relief has been established. Certain psychiatric disorders have been associated with nutritional factors, and barring the presence of dangerous or incapacitating symptoms, those factors should always be addressed first. Laying the appropriate nutritional groundwork via dietary interventions and/or supplements, which varies by diagnosis, prior to or concurrently with medications is likely a sound approach. This includes supplying adequate amounts of required nutrients for neurotransmitter production, maintaining cellular membranes, and addressing dysfunction in the IIO axis.

NBP protocols for various psychiatric disorders are works in progress and will undoubtedly be modified based on the availability of additional research. The following approach has been found to be effective for the management of psychiatric conditions, including mood, anxiety, psychotic, and developmental disorders. It's common sense that ingested food and chemicals directly affect a person's biochemistry, health, and mental functions.

In most cases, diet is not likely to be the sole cause of psychiatric conditions. However, by addressing core targets of essential nutrient availability, the IIO axis, and membrane function, optimizing certain dietary factors can influence the presentation, severity, and comorbidities associated with them. Put simply, the intent is to increase nutrient-dense foods while minimizing toxins and allergens. Approaching this process with the absolutes of "never" or "always" seems to be less helpful than using the relative terms of "increasing" or "decreasing" certain elements in the diet. Refer to Table 4.

Table 4: General Guidelines for Eating to Optimize Mental and General Health

Increase Intake of foods that are...	Decrease Intake of...
-Fresh	-Foods with preservatives
-Organic*	-Foods grown with pesticides
-Sprouted	-Flour that is milled weeks and months prior to consumption
-Raw	-Processed, overcooked, and deep-fried foods
-Grass/forage fed and free range	-Grain/feedlot fed and caged animals
-Wild (fish and game)	-Farmed fish
-High in ORAC** value	-Foods with artificial sweeteners, colors, and flavors
-High in live probiotic cultures***	-Suspected and known food allergens

*Choosing organic foods ensures that there are no pesticide residues on or in your food. The Environmental Working Group puts out an annual list of foods with the most and least pesticides at https://www.ewg.org/foodnews/index.php The group estimates that individuals can reduce their exposure to pesticides by 80% if they just avoid certain nonorganic foods.

**Oxygen radical absorbance capacity (ORAC) is a measure of antioxidant capacity of food in vitro. Fresh fruits and vegetables tend to have higher ORAC values than preserved and cooked foods do.

***Probiotic-rich foods include sauerkraut, kimchi, yogurt, kefir, kvass, kombucha, miso, pickled vegetables, etc. Look for these foods in the refrigerated section and for indications on the labels that the product contains *live cultures*.

Models for Using NBP

NBP may be implemented in several different ways, depending upon the clinical situation. In general, NBP may be used in a comprehensive, targeted, or complementary fashion. After assessment, these approaches all start with identifying and addressing nutritional deficiencies associated with the client's diagnosis. This involves ordering blood work, followed by dietary and/or supplement interventions and follow-up laboratory tests to demonstrate correction.

After these initial steps, the comprehensive approach uses essential nutrients prescribed concurrently, followed by serial trials of metabolic nutrients, and lastly, serial trials of herbal interventions. The targeted approach of NBP uses selective interventions in a serial manner from any category most likely to be safe and effective in addressing the client's specific symptoms. Complementary use of NBP refers to selective interventions used along with prescription medications likely to improve the efficacy of the medication, allow for a reduced dose of the medication, and/or address residual symptoms and adverse effects of the medication.

A number of factors determine which NBP model is most appropriate to use in various situations. Initially, severity of illness, patient preference, and treatment naïveté are taken into account. Those with highly debilitating conditions commonly require interventions with prescription psychotropics to reduce symptom severity rapidly and achieve stability *prior* to using NBP.

Client Preference
A client often enters psychiatric treatment with a preference for a certain form of intervention. On the extreme are those who would prefer to avoid any synthetic interventions at all costs versus those who only want prescription medications because they feel that these are the only "real" medicines that work. Past treatment history can range from none to multiple trials of medications and supplements with varying degrees of success and side effects. Once treatment is under way, compliance with medications and/or supplements, efficacy, and adverse events largely guide the course. The comprehensive use of NBP

requires the consumption of multiple (usually five or more) supplements daily. A certain degree of willingness and organization on the client's part is necessary for success. It helps to make it clear at the outset that the regimen starts with a few essential supplements and grows slowly over time.

Case Study A

A man in his mid-30s was diagnosed with ADHD inattentive subtype as an adult but had never been assessed as a child; he was also diagnosed with significant symptoms of social anxiety. For a number of years, he drank up to two large glasses of wine per night but felt that it worsened his ADHD symptoms. He also reported a long-standing history of poor digestion and constipation. Food sensitivity testing revealed delayed reactions to dairy, gluten, egg whites, coffee, beets, and several other foods, which when removed from his diet improved his digestion and constipation. He had been prescribed a delayed-release stimulant medication that improved his symptoms but also caused insomnia. He later tried atomoxetine, which was effective but caused constipation.

At evaluation, he reported that he had been taking a comprehensive nutrient formula with a vast array of ingredients. The supplements included essential vitamins, minerals, fatty acids, probiotics, metabolic nutrients, and herbs; some had evidence for treating ADHD symptoms, but many did not.

Evidence-based metabolic supplements and herbs the client was taking upon presentation:

Phosphatidylserine: 33mg

Acetyl-L-carnitine: 150mg

N-acetyl-L-cysteine: 74mg

S-adenosylmethionine (SAMe): 200mg

L-tyrosine: 300mg

Pine bark extract (pycnogenol): 50mg

Bacopa: 300mg

Ginkgo extract: 250mg

Gotu kola extract: 225mg

Passionflower extract: 90mg

As can be seen, his doses of phosphatidylserine (PS), acetyl-L-carnitine (ALCAR), N-acetylcysteine (NAC), and pycnogenol were below the doses found to be effective in addressing ADHD symptoms. Essential nutrients were adequately addressed, so laboratory tests were not likely to be necessary. As it was impossible to determine what effect, if any, each component of this multinutrient blend was having, I suggested discontinuing the overly inclusive combination, and we replaced it with a basic multivitamin and 1500-2000mg of EPA, optimized the probiotic he was taking, added magnesium citrate (weight based), and titrated his dose of PS up to 400mg twice per day.

After a few weeks, he reported improved control of ADHD symptoms, but anxiety was still an issue. Theanine was added and titrated to 200mg twice per day and 200mg at bedtime. This resulted in improved anxiety symptoms and improved sleep. Psychotherapy was also implemented with a focus on the etiology (the origins or causes of a disease) and manifestations of his anxiety symptoms.

This client was quite motivated to attain even better control of his symptoms, so ALCAR and NAC were each tried as a monotherapy added to essential supplements, and each had a therapeutic effect on his ADHD symptoms. He chose to take two out of three of these metabolic supplements at a time in addition to essential nutrients and rotated them every two to three weeks: NAC 600mg twice per day, ALCAR 1000mg in the morning, and PS 400mg in the morning and 300mg in the early afternoon.

We discussed an NBP approach to anxiety and occasional insomnia, which could also address ADHD symptoms. Lemon balm, valerian, and the amino acid tryptophan were tried at various times, each having desired therapeutic effects; the lemon balm also significantly improved his cognitive performance. These supplements were taken at bedtime on a rotating basis.

For more than one year, taking this combination of supplements, as well as avoiding foods for which he had intolerance, pesticides, and additives has provided an effective treatment of ADHD symptoms recognized by the client and his family. Symptoms of social anxiety have also been addressed with a combination of supplements and psychotherapy.

This case illustrates successful treatment of both ADHD and anxiety symptoms with an NBP approach coupled with psychotherapy. The client desired this form of intervention after having some success with prescription medication but experiencing side effects while taking them. He displayed high levels of motivation and organization, which translated into not only taking a complex regimen of supplements daily but also exercising regularly, being mindful of his diet, and working on issues in psychotherapy.

Obstacles to Compliance

Obstacles to compliance may include keeping supplements stocked, opening multiple bottles daily (weekly pillboxes are helpful), difficulty swallowing pills, and experiencing adverse events. Clients who prefer avoiding prescription medications and who would like to keep their daily pill count to a minimum do better with a more targeted approach. When supplements alone are ineffective or partially effective, prescription medications can be added to target outstanding symptoms and vice versa.

The following is an example of how NBP may be used comprehensively for the treatment of ADHD:

1. After appropriate evaluation for the presence and subtype of ADHD, as well as comorbid conditions, assess the need for immediate intervention with prescription medication, including serious academic and behavioral difficulties that require rapid symptom relief. In such cases, it may be necessary to recommend starting treatment with a first-line FDA-approved medication for ADHD.

2. Identify any nutritional deficiencies associated with ADHD, including deficiencies in magnesium, zinc, iron, and omega-3 fats, during psychiatric assessment. If such deficiencies are present, address them with dietary modifications and/or supplements.

3. Next, add a broad-spectrum essential-nutrient approach, composed of specific suggestions for dietary modifications and a multivitamin-mineral supplement, along with specific omega-3 fats and probiotics. It can take from several weeks to two months to assess whether these essential nutrient interventions have had clinical benefit. If necessary, trials of metabolic supplements may occur serially to determine the effects of each; effective or partially effective interventions may then be combined or cycled. Herbs may also be

used serially in a similar fashion. When necessary, medications can be prescribed for residual symptoms.

4. Finally, adjust supplements and medications and monitor laboratory test values during the maintenance and follow-up phase of treatment.

Why NBP?

If a nutritional approach can be therapeutic, why aren't psychiatrists recommending it more often? An article in the *Nutrition Journal* suggests that doctors primarily resist using supplements as treatments because of their lack of knowledge.[42] Understandably, many psychiatrists may have a sense of safety from knowing that a medication prescribed for a condition is approved and monitored by the FDA.[43] The mental health insurance industry also influences prescribing practices by tending to treat inpatient and outpatient psychiatric services that involve prescription medications as more payable.

In fact, on inpatient units, medications must often be started or adjusted every few days in order to "justify" the stay. Care must be taken that the practice of psychiatry considers important aspects of neurofunctioning and the aforementioned therapeutic targets while incorporating the use of pharmaceuticals. In many cases, doctors may consider prescribing nutritional interventions but only after medications don't provide sufficient relief or have negative side effects. All too often, treatment becomes fragmented among the doctor's prescription medication approach and other nonmedical providers who are addressing nutritional and supplement issues. The relative lack of knowledge about one another's disciplines is not optimal for patient care.

Physician Education

Although evidence for using nutritional therapies to treat psychiatric conditions is limited when compared with that for pharmaceuticals, numerous well-designed studies indicate that such interventions can be safe and effective. The evidence includes correlations between nutritional status and mental illness, multinutrient, single-nutrient, and adjunctive studies.

Nutritional interventions can compensate for both deficiencies and excesses in the diet; the shortcomings of modern food production; and metabolic differences due to genetic, age, and environmental factors. It may be preferable to address psychiatric disorders exclusively or adjunctively with naturally occurring substances the body is familiar with rather than introducing novel foreign chemicals; in many cases, these naturally occurring substances have become essential over long periods of evolutionary time.

When an abundance of data indicates that a nutritional approach to treating a medical disorder is effective, the supplement may be *medicinalized*, meaning it is marketed to the public and/or physicians in a way that resembles the marketing of a prescription medication. An example of this is methylfolate (MF), which is the methylated (activated) form of the vitamin folic acid. Because of the accumulated evidence that MF may be effective in the treatment of depression, a "medical food" was marketed that contained high-dose MF. A *medical food* is "a food formulated to be consumed or administered enterally (orally) under the supervision of a physician and is intended for the specific dietary management of a disease or condition for which distinctive nutritional requirements, based on recognized scientific principles, are established by medical evaluation."[44]

In essence, the intent was to turn a vitamin, available in high-dose forms from multiple manufacturers, into a physician-endorsed treatment for depression. It helps to educate physicians about an effective nutritional intervention for depression and increases its use by patients who are suffering. This same principle may be applied to a number of other effective nutrients as laid out in NBP.

It is clear that educating physicians about nutritional treatment options is an important task that cannot be ignored. Doing so will help a significant number of patients who do not respond adequately or have untoward side effects from prescription medications. Education may also provide physician-endorsed avenues of relief to patients suffering from psychiatric conditions who are noncompliant with medications.[45]

Client Education
The efficacy of nutritional interventions in psychiatry and general health, underuse of it by doctors, and the growing consumer demand create the need for an evidence-based, systematic medium physicians can integrate into their practices. Many patients also want a way to communicate their desires clearly in a format that can be easily understood and implemented. NBP is an attempt to provide such a medium for clients to use with their physicians. What follows is how NBP can be specifically applied to the treatment of ADHD.

Chapter 7

Guide to Integrating Nutrient-Based Psychiatry® into the Medical Management of ADHD

NPB addresses the overall health of the client. It is now known that the majority of psychiatric disorders are associated with oxidative stress, inflammation, immune system dysfunction, and/or membrane lipid abnormalities. These factors also underlie most medical illnesses, many of which occur comorbidly with some psychiatric conditions. Virtually all interventions used in NBP have antioxidant, anti-inflammatory, immunomodulating, and/or membrane-lipid therapy properties. The ability to regulate these key systems may be partly responsible for their therapeutic benefits, may address or prevent comorbid conditions, and benefits the patient's overall health status.

ADHD Causes and Correlation

ADHD has high heterogeneity with regard to presentation and etiology. Essentially, it is a disorder that may present in several different ways depending upon the combination of underlying causes.

When considering the cause(s) of ADHD or any other medical or psychiatric disorder, for that matter, understanding the relationship between correlation and causation can help avoid confusion. Evidence for the causes of a disorder is often initially based on correlational data. After a sufficient amount of empirical observation, two or more variables may be found to correlate with one another. This does not necessarily mean that one variable has caused the other. Rather, correlation is a necessary finding and may be seen as an indicator for causation, but it, alone, does not constitute sufficient proof of the cause.

Once correlation is established, systematically exploring every possible causational relationship to rule out other possibilities, including coincidence and the existence of other unknown variables that may be causative, is required. Often, the interrelationships between large numbers of variables in biological systems can be so complex that causation is quite difficult to determine.

The current understanding is that there is no single cause of ADHD. It does have high heritability, but that does not rule out contributions from environmental factors owing to gene-environment interactions. Environmental factors may be mediated by genetic factors and vice versa.[46] The genetic contribution to ADHD is multigenetic[47] and appears to be explained by a complex blend of common and rare genetic variants.[48] There is a large network of small genetic variations that behave additively and interact to produce a disruption of neural architecture behaviorally expressed in the core symptoms of ADHD.[49] A number of environmental factors have been correlated with ADHD, many of which are seen as risk factors. Prenatal and perinatal factors include maternal smoking and alcohol and substance abuse, maternal stress, low birth weight, and prematurity. Although they are considered to be risk factors, causality has not been proven.

Exposure to environmental toxins, such as pesticides, polychlorinated biphenyl (PCB), and lead, is also correlated with ADHD, and although these toxins are seen as risk factors, they are not considered to be causative. Nutritional deficiencies (zinc, magnesium, essential fatty acids) and surpluses (sugar and artificial food colorings) are correlated with ADHD but are not considered to be risk factors. Family adversity, low income, familial conflict, and parent-child hostility are correlated but are not considered to be risk factors. Severe early deprivation is correlated, considered to be a risk factor, and is likely causative of ADHD.[50]

Given the complex multifactorial etiology and the different presentations, it is best to treat ADHD with a circumspect approach. This type of approach supplies the best chance of addressing the possible underlying causes, risk factors, and associated conditions, rather than simply treating the symptoms.

ADHD Research and the Placebo Effect

In medicine, results from clinical trials are used to determine whether an intervention is effective in treating a condition. Results from double-blind placebo-controlled trials produce the highest quality data that can be used when making clinical decisions. In these types of trials, participants with similar characteristics are randomly assigned to receive either an active intervention or a placebo, which is essentially a fake or inactive treatment. When both participants and administrators of the treatment do not know who receives the actual treatment and who receives the placebo, this is known as a *double-blind study*. The *placebo effect* refers to the sham treatment improving a patient's condition because there is an expectation that it will be helpful. Placebo response rates can vary depending on many factors, including the condition being studied, the nature of the relationship between the investigator and patient, and characteristics of the placebo, as well as the population being studied.

Such population characteristics include the age of the participants. Preliminary conclusions of literature reviews and meta-analyses of data indicate that placebo rates are higher in children and adolescents than in adults, but drug response rates are similar. In general, age is negatively correlated with the size of the placebo response, so studies on younger children may have the greatest placebo effect. This has been observed particularly in children with depression. These findings suggest that in studies investigating the effects of interventions on children and adolescents, a greater number of participants is needed to achieve significance in the data than would be needed for adult studies, and the efficacy of the placebo should be assessed not only against interventions that are assumed to be more effective but also against no intervention. In clinical trials on response rates to ADHD treatment, placebos were effective 20% to 30% of the time in children[51] as opposed to a 10% response rate in adults.[52] Therefore, caution must be used when making clinical decisions based on data from randomized controlled trials in children with ADHD.

Oxidative Stress and ADHD

Multiple lines of evidence suggest an association between oxidative stress and ADHD. Metabolic markers of oxidative stress are significantly altered in patients with ADHD.[53] These markers can include oxidative DNA damage; malondialdehyde (MDA), an end product of lipid peroxidation; exhaled ethane, a marker of increased oxidative breakdown of omega-3 fats; nitric oxide, a *pro-oxidant*, which is a substance that accelerates the oxidation of another substance; superoxide dismutase, an endogenous antioxidant; total oxidative status; and oxidative stress index. A recently published meta-analysis examined the association between ADHD and oxidative stress in 231 medication-naïve ADHD patients and 207 controls. Findings suggest that persons with ADHD have normal levels of antioxidant production, but their responses to oxidative stress may be insufficient and lead to increased oxidative damage.[54]

Moreover, MDA levels have been correlated with the presence and severity of ADHD symptoms in adults, number of ADHD criteria met ($p<0.01$), and elevations in total hyperactivity/impulsivity scores ($p<0.02$).[55] Total oxidative status, an index or estimate of the level of oxidative stress in a biological system, was found to be so consistently elevated in adults with ADHD that it may be used as a predictive indicator for the diagnosis, with an 86% positive predictive value and 100% negative predictive value.[56] This means that 86% of the time, if a subject's total oxidative status is elevated to a certain level, the person meets the criteria for ADHD; and 100% of the time that it is not elevated, the person does *not* have ADHD. However, studies investigating the correlation between ADHD and MDA levels in children have produced contradictory results.[57,58,59]

It appears that the metabolism of the catecholamine neurotransmitters (epinephrine, norepinephrine, and dopamine) is dysregulated in patients with ADHD.[60] A likely source of the associated oxidative stress is greater synthesis and breakdown (turnover) of catecholamines. At high concentrations, the metabolism of these neurotransmitters forms superoxide and hydroxyl-free radicals, leading to exhaustion of endogenous antioxidants with subsequent DNA, lipid, and protein damage; the increased metabolism of catecholamine neurotransmitters directly leads to increased oxidative stress, which may further compound ADHD symptom presentation. Given the weight of these findings, the therapeutic role of antioxidants in ADHD has been discussed and explored in recent years.[61]

Stimulant Medications and Antioxidants

Prescription stimulant medications, such as methylphenidate and amphetamines that are commonly used to treat ADHD, may have pro-oxidant[62] effects. When abused, they may also contribute to inflammation[63] and decreased levels of endogenous antioxidants.[64] There is evidence that antioxidants may play a role against amphetamine-induced cellular dysfunction.[65] These findings imply that some of the deleterious effects of prescription medications may be countered by consuming higher levels of certain antioxidants.

Melatonin is a hormone and supplement that scavenges free radicals and stimulates the production of endogenous antioxidants. It may decrease amphetamine-induced toxicity, nerve degeneration, immunoreactivity, and elevated levels of alpha-synuclein (a neuronal protein involved in neurodegenerative disorders).[66] Similarly, N-acetylcysteine (NAC), a potent antioxidant supplement, may protect against amphetamine-induced oxidative protein damage.[67] However, animal studies implicating stimulant medications in oxidative stress were performed on healthy animals (not ADHD animal models), as opposed to human subjects with ADHD who were taking therapeutic doses of stimulant medications. In an in vitro study examining the effects of methamphetamine, methylphenidate, and atomoxetine, no cytotoxic (cell toxicity) effects were found at concentrations that would be therapeutic in treating ADHD.[68]

Interestingly, these medications significantly enhanced cell survival in human neuronal and immune cells. Given the potential detrimental effects of stimulant medications on biological systems, these findings are surprising but may be related to stimulants' effects on cocaine- and amphetamine-regulated transcript peptide, which may be neuroprotective via preservation of mitochondrial function or upregulation of brain-derived neurotrophic factor, mRNA expression, and protein synthesis.[69] Additionally, there is evidence that when prescribed at therapeutic doses for pediatric clients with ADHD, stimulant medications may promote the maturation process in areas of the brain that commonly lag behind in this population.[70]

Magnetic resonance imaging studies comparing brain volumes of stimulant-naïve children with ADHD with those treated long term with stimulants and a neurotypical control group have shown that the stimulant-naïve group had significantly smaller brain volumes in a number of different areas than did the other two groups. This fact suggests that long-term use of therapeutic-level stimulants to treat ADHD may normalize the volumes of some brain areas.

To summarize, ADHD has been closely associated with a number of markers of increased oxidative stress, which may be related to dysregulation of catecholamine metabolism. Stimulant medications often used to treat ADHD may have pro-oxidant, neurotoxic, and inflammatory effects, but, when given at therapeutic doses to clients with ADHD, stimulants may be neuroprotective and neurocorrective morphologically.

Improving the overall antioxidant status in clients with ADHD would mitigate the increased oxidative stress associated with the condition, as well as possible harmful effects posed by prescribed stimulant medications. Thus far, there is some limited evidence that addressing oxidative stress in ADHD is correlated with clinical improvements.[71] Over time, antioxidant therapy may prove to be an effective first-line intervention for the treatment for ADHD.

Allergic Hypersensitivity and ADHD

A subset of cases of ADHD may be caused or exacerbated by allergic responses. An *allergy* is a hypersensitivity disorder of the immune system, occurring when the system reacts to substances in the environment, such as certain foods, pollens, dust, etc. Allergic inflammation is a feature of several allergy-associated medical conditions, including allergic rhinitis (AR), allergic asthma, and atopic dermatitis. AR is characterized by nasal congestion, runny nose, itchy and watery eyes, sneezing, snoring and mouth breathing, postnasal drip, and yellow-green nasal discharge.

Sleep Disorders from Allergies

Collectively, these AR symptoms may lead to nocturnal microarousals (brief awakenings) and sleep fragmentation[72] that results in sleep loss, daytime fatigue, learning impairment,[73] and decreased cognitive function,[74] resembling the core symptoms of ADHD.[75] AR and breathing-related sleep problems are significantly associated with ADHD.[76] The authors of an article in *SLEEP* concluded that 81% of children with ADHD who habitually snore could have their ADHD symptoms eliminated if the snoring and other breathing-related sleep disorders were effectively treated; overall, this group represents 25% of all children with ADHD.[77] Therefore, it is important to assess for these conditions because they affect a potentially large percentage of patients.

Food Allergies

Adverse reactions to food or food components may be associated with behavioral disturbances in ADHD.[78] This includes pesticides[79] and artificial food colorings, flavorings, and preservatives.[80] When ADHD symptoms develop in response to foods or food components and immunological mechanisms are identified, ADHD is a consequence of an allergic response.[81] As a contributing factor to ADHD symptoms, a food or food-components allergy is best determined by means of oral provocation tests or improvement during an avoidance test or elimination diet.[82]

It has been hypothesized that persons with ADHD may fall into two distinct populations: hypersensitive, or allergic, ADHD and nonhypersensitive, or nonallergic, ADHD.[83] Identifying and avoiding allergic triggers (in both food and the environment) in susceptible clients decreases the predisposition for ADHD symptoms and reduces the need for other interventions.

PART THREE: TREATING ADHD WITH NUTRIENT-BASED PSYCHIATRY®

Part Three is written specifically for the psychiatrists and other medical professionals who treat ADHD. The remainder of this book includes specific treatment strategies intended to be implemented by physicians and psychiatrists in a standard medical format, including data on efficacy, adverse events, medication and nutrient interactions, pharmacodynamics, carcinogenicity, effects on fertility, and use in pregnancy and lactation.

In this way, these strategies may be seen as acceptable and viable for clinical integration by physicians. Please remember that this text represents just one doctor's opinion and experiences with using nutritional interventions to treat psychiatric disorders. Alternative interpretations and implementations of the evidence are possible. When compared with FDA-approved first-line treatments for ADHD, this approach has limited evidence.

Chapter 8

Pharmacological Targets for Treating ADHD

In medicine, *biochemical* (meaning medicinal and supplemental) interventions target various aspects of human metabolism in order to produce a therapeutic response, ideally with limited or no adverse effects. The following is a review of current pharmacological targets that might be effective in addressing causes and symptoms of ADHD.

Catecholamines

Catecholamines are a class of NTs, consisting of dopamine (DA), norepinephrine (NE), and epinephrine (E). The former two are well-established targets for the majority of prescription medications for ADHD, including methylphenidate, amphetamines, atomoxetine, and bupropion,[84] as well as several interventions used in NBP. Although there may be greater turnover of these NTs in those with ADHD, insufficient production of catecholamines, specifically in the prefrontal cortex (a brain area associated with planning complex cognitive behaviors and executive function), has been implicated.

Because stimulants are highly effective at increasing NE and DA in this area of the brain, they are thought to address core symptoms of ADHD[85] successfully, with estimates ranging from 56% to 85%.[86] This class of medications exerts it effects on catecholamines more effectively than naturally occurring interventions do. Approximately 10% to 30% of clients do not respond to stimulants or may experience adverse effects, including appetite suppression, sleep disturbances, mood lability, and exacerbation of tics.[87]

Serotonin

Serotonin, also known as *5-hydroxytryptamine (5-HT)*, is a neurotransmitter derived from the amino acid tryptophan.

Its functions are thought to include the regulation of mood, sleep, and appetite and the cognitive functions of memory and learning. In psychiatry, medications that modulate the metabolism of 5-HT are commonly prescribed for symptoms of depression and anxiety. Evidence suggests that aberrations in the metabolism of 5-HT may be related to symptoms of ADHD. 5-HT may regulate hyperactivity and impulsivity and affect dopaminergic transmission.[88] Despite some contradictory evidence,[89] preliminary investigations requiring additional follow-up studies to determine reproducibility indicate that 5-HT levels and/or activity in those with ADHD may be decreased.[90,91,92,93,94,95] Changes in 5-HT metabolism in those with ADHD may be due, in part, to variations in associated genes that affect 5-HT transporters, metabolism, and receptor sites.[96] Candidate gene analyses have shown modest but significant associations between the presence of ADHD and these single gene variants.[97,98,99,100,101] It has been hypothesized that when multiple genetic markers are considered in tandem, the effect on development of ADHD may be highly significant.[102] Although scant evidence suggests that the SSRI medication fluoxetine is effective in treating ADHD symptoms,[103,104] further well-controlled studies are required for confirmation. Given the current evidence linking 5-HT with ADHD, it is curious that there have not been additional investigations into the therapeutic use of serotonergic medications and supplements. The mainstay of conventional ADHD treatment, the psychostimulants, act mainly adrenergically. For reasons that remain unclear, 5-HT has an important role in potentiating their therapeutic effect.[105]

Acetylcholine (Ach)

Ach is a neurotransmitter associated with arousal, reward, sustained attention, memory, learning, and behavior. Recently, evidence has been emerging that dysfunction or deficits of this neurotransmitter system (also known as *cholinergic*) may be related to the pathophysiology of ADHD; this may be especially true of the combined subtype of ADHD.[106] Moreover, nicotinic

Ach receptor function has been associated with impulsivity,[107] and there are preliminary findings that boys with ADHD may have decreased muscarinic Ach receptor density.[108] Polymorphisms in the genes that code for choline transporters[109] and the alpha 4 subunit of the nicotinic Ach receptor[110] have been associated with ADHD. Therefore, cholinergic agonist therapy has been proposed as a mechanism to treat ADHD symptoms.[111]

Nicotinic Ach receptor agonists have demonstrated significant efficacy in this regard in adult populations.[112] Donepezil, an acetylcholinesterase inhibitor that blocks the deactivation of Ach, may be effective in treating children with ADHD[113] and ADHD-like symptoms in case series reports.[114] However, in a randomized controlled pilot study, galantamine (another Ach inhibitor) failed to show efficacy for adults with ADHD when administered at doses used for the treatment of Alzheimer's dementia.[115] Given the evidence, it may follow that interventions addressing cholinergic dysfunction could be therapeutic for a subpopulation of ADHD clients who have cholinergic deficits, possibly related to genetic differences.

Glutamate (Glu)

Glutamate is a primary excitatory neurotransmitter in the central nervous system (CNS) with several receptor types, including N-methyl-D-aspartate (NMDA), alpha-amino-3-hydroxy-5-methyl-4-isoxazolepropionic acid (AMPA), and metabotropic receptors. Mounting evidence suggests that glutamatergic transmission may be dysregulated in ADHD. Genetic studies indicate that polymorphisms and copy number variants in genes coding for glutamate receptors are significantly associated with the presence of ADHD.[116] One study found that autoantibodies against glutamic acid decarboxylase, one of the enzymes that converts glutamate to gamma-aminobutyric acid (GABA), which is a major inhibitory neurotransmitter in the CNS, were found in 27% of subjects with ADHD but not in controls.[117]

If present in a subset of clients with ADHD, these antibodies binding to GAD decrease enzymatic activity, leading to increased levels of glutamate and decreased synthesis and release of GABA. Decreased levels of GABA have been observed in ADHD. Investigations on animal models of ADHD indicate that glutamate is increased.[118] Spectroscopy studies provide evidence of increased ratios of glutamate in several brain areas.[119] This has been observed in children and adolescents with ADHD who more often have a combined type of presentation (with hyperactivity) as opposed to adults who more commonly have the inattentive subtype. Collateral information shows positive correlations between impulsivity and glutamate levels.[120]

Treating ADHD with stimulant medications, as well as the nonstimulant, atomoxetine, commonly results in decreased (normalized) glutamate ratios on spectroscopic scans.[121] The complex reciprocal relationships between activation levels of dopamine and glutamate receptor subtypes have clinical relevance for the treatment of ADHD. In general, as dopaminergic receptor activity increases, glutamatergic activity tends to decrease. This may, in part, explain why elevated glutamate levels are observed in untreated combined type ADHD and dopaminergic medications have been associated with decreased glutamate levels and symptom improvement. Interventions aimed at decreasing glutamatergic tone may be therapeutic in ADHD.

Indeed, atomoxetine, in addition to increasing catecholamine levels has been found to antagonize NMDA receptors, an action that may account for some of its clinical efficacy.[122] Two small open-label trials provide evidence that memantine, an NMDA receptor antagonist indicated for Alzheimer's dementia, may be safe and effective in the treatment of ADHD in adults and children.[123] Recent preliminary animal and human studies suggest that a medication amplifying the effects of glutamate at the AMPA receptor site is effective in treating adult ADHD.[124] It may follow that interventions used in NBP that modulate glutamate activity, including phosphatidylserine, N-acetylcysteine, L-the-anine, and magnesium, could also benefit clients with ADHD.

Gamma-Aminobutyric Acid (GABA)

This is a primary inhibitory neurotransmitter in the CNS. Manip-ulation of GABA levels and receptor sites are common targets for many pharmaceuticals and natural agents. Animal data reflect that impulsivity is associated with significantly lower GABA receptor binding in the anterior cingulate cortex.[125] Spec-troscopic evidence indicates that levels of GABA are decreased in the primary somatosensory and motor cortices of children with ADHD when compared with those of controls.[126]

Furthermore, increased levels of GABA in the prefrontal cortex are correlated with decreased urgency, one aspect of impul-sivity.[127] As discussed, GABA and glutamate have a reciprocal relationship, and antibodies against the enzyme that converts glutamate to GABA were seen in 27% of an ADHD cohort.[128] GABAergic modulating interventions could conceivably be ther-apeutic in the treatment of ADHD. Unfortunately, with regard to direct clinical application of GABAergic pharmaceuticals, very little information exists in the literature. However, several natural interventions that modulate GABA, including vitamin B6, magnesium, lemon balm, and passionflower, have some preliminary evidence for efficacy.

Oxidative Stress and Membrane-Lipid Therapy

Several markers of increased oxidative stress are associated with the presence of ADHD. Improvement of some of these has been correlated with symptom improvement. This is a target that often goes largely unaddressed by conventional treat-ment. A number of interventions used in NBP for ADHD are anti-oxidants, such as acetyl-L-carnitine, N-acetylcysteine, pycnog-enol, phosphatidylserine, and omega-3 fats. When antioxidant interventions specifically target lipid oxidation, they may also be considered a form of membrane-lipid therapy.

As previously discussed, the constituents of the membrane are another important therapeutic target. This is addressed mainly by phosphatidylserine, omega-3 fats, and antioxidants that prevent lipid peroxidation.

Genetically and Nutritionally Influenced Pathways of Synthesis and Metabolism of Neurotransmitters

Genetic variations and availability of certain essential nutrients like amino acids, B vitamins, and minerals can impair the metabolism of neurotransmitters implicated in ADHD. Maintaining an adequate supply of raw materials and ensuring potentially sluggish enzymes are supersaturated may be an effective approach to treating ADHD.

Allergic Hypersensitivity, Inflammation, and Immune Effects

A subset of ADHD cases may be primarily driven by allergic hypersensitivity. Allergens in the environment, along with their adverse inflammatory and immune effects, can create or exacerbate the presentation of ADHD. There are both pharmaceutical and nutritional approaches designed to address this.

Chapter 9

Treating ADHD with NBP
Phase I: Assessment

The initial step in addressing ADHD is screening and evaluation. These processes have been described by the American Academy of Child and Adolescent Psychiatry most recently in 2007.[129] Regardless of the chief complaint, questions about the presence and severity of inattention, impulsivity, and hyperactivity are posed. Rating scales that contain the *Diagnostic and Statistical Manual of Mental Disorders* (DSM) symptoms of ADHD[130] could be included in the initial screening. If parents or clients report that ADHD symptoms are present and causing impairment, a full evaluation of ADHD is warranted. This process involves clinical interviews with parents and patients; the use of ADHD symptom rating scales (completed by parents, teachers, and patients); and obtaining a detailed psychiatric family history and perinatal, developmental, medical, and past psychiatric history. Certain medical conditions and historical elements such as history of head injury, lead and fetal alcohol exposure, encephalopathies, and hyperthyroidism may require additional laboratory and/or neurological investigations. If the patient's history is suggestive of low general cognitive ability or low achievement in language or mathematics relative to intellectual ability, psychological and neuropsychological tests should be performed to determine whether learning disorders are present. In most cases, such tests are not mandatory for the diagnosis of ADHD.

In addition to standard psychiatric evaluation for presence of an ADHD diagnosis and subtype, it is imperative to assess for certain comorbid conditions that may exacerbate or even be causative of ADHD symptoms. Their detection and management are critical in the circumspect treatment of ADHD. Comorbidities that may be associated with ADHD include oppositional defiant disorder, conduct disorder, antisocial personality disorder (in adults), substance abuse, anxiety, and mood[131] and sleep disorders.

Sleep Disorders

An estimated 25% to 50% of children with ADHD struggle with sleep problems, including instability of sleep onset, increased latency, bedtime resistance, nighttime awakenings, restlessness during sleep, difficulty awakening, and sleep duration.[132] In fact, these findings are so consistent that sleep measures alone can significantly predict whether a child has a diagnosis of ADHD.[133] Poor sleep adversely affects the prefrontal cortex, potentially impairing the executive functioning necessary for attention and emotional regulation, resulting in symptoms that resemble ADHD. A subset of ADHD cases may be exacerbated by sleep difficulties.

Stimulant medications used in ADHD are significantly associated with difficulty initiating or maintaining sleep.[134] The well-documented interplay between allergic rhinitis (AR) and other breathing-related sleep disorders and ADHD symptoms was discussed in an earlier chapter. Therefore, a thorough assessment of both breathing- and nonbreathing-related sleep disorders associated with ADHD is warranted.

Allergic Rhinitis (AR) and Breathing-Related Sleep Disorders
Ask about the following symptoms in conjunction with sleep disturbance:

Nasal congestion

Runny nose

Itchy and watery eyes

Sneezing

Snoring and mouth breathing

Postnasal drip

Yellow-green nasal discharge

If there are significant positive findings, refer the client to an allergist; ear, nose, and throat specialist; or primary care physician for treatment. Additionally, probiotics, pycnogenol, and spirulina, which are discussed later in this text, may have therapeutic effects.

Nonbreathing-Related Sleep Disorders
Ask about the following aspects of sleep. If significant symptoms are present, address them with suggested NBP or conventional approaches.

Increased sleep latency

Middle insomnia (awakening in the night)

Early-morning awakening

Total sleep time

Naps

Difficulty waking up in the morning

Sleep that does not feel restful and restorative

Excessive nocturnal movements (waking up in an entirely different position with the covers and pillows displaced)

Dietary Assessment
In order to get a sense of the client's and his or her family's dietary habits, ask specific questions about the consumption of the following:

Breakfast, lunch, dinner, and snacks on school days and weekends

Fast foods

Sugars: soda, sweets, flour, and other processed carbohydrates

Caffeine: coffee, tea, soda, energy drinks, chocolate

Organic foods

Fresh fruits and vegetables

Proteins: meats, fish, dairy, eggs, grass- or forage-fed animals

Fats: vegetable oils, salad dressings, fried foods, partially hydrogenated oils (snack cakes, cake mixes, frostings, dough-nuts, some types of peanut butter, fish sticks, margarine and shortening, microwave popcorn, noodles, frozen foods)

Artificial food colorings (candy, sports drinks, sodas, snack foods, breakfast cereals)

Also inquire about known or suspected food allergies and intol-erances and how they were determined.

Recommended Laboratory Tests

The following laboratory tests are recommended during the evaluation period:

Red blood cell (RBC) omega-6:omega-3 ratio (n-6:n-3): This is a test that most laboratories do not perform and most insur-ance plans do not cover. If the test is not financially feasible, empirical treatment with omega-3 fats is still recommended. When obtained, the test provides objective data about what is happening in cell membranes with regard to omega-6 and omega-3 status. A repeat value obtained three to six months into treatment with n-3 fats and dietary interventions aimed at decreasing n-6 intake may be correlated with symptom improvement. This test costs between $130 and $300 and is available from Genova Labs and a number of online retailers that sell home testing kits.

RBC Mg: Because only 1% of the magnesium in the body is extra-cellular, doing a standard electrolyte panel will not provide much information about what is happening intracellularly with regard to magnesium status. Again, most laboratories do not perform this test, and most insurance does not cover it. If the test is not financially feasible, empirical treatment with magnesium is still recommended. As was the case with n-6:n-3 ratio, repeating the RBC Mg test three to six months into treatment with Mg supplements may indicate correlation with symptom improvement. This test costs between $100 and $200 and is available from Genova and other laboratories.

Serum or plasma zinc: This is a widely available laboratory test. If values are low and supplementation occurs as part of treatment, the test may be repeated three to six months later, and values may correlate with symptom improvement.

Ferritin: This test indicates the amount of stored iron in the body and is widely available. If values are low and treatment is initiated in the form of iron supplements, the test may be repeated in three to six months, and values may correlate with symptom improvement.

Vitamin D: This test is ordered as "25-hydroxyvitamin D" and is widely available. If values are low and treatment is initiated, the test may be repeated after three months.

Chapter 10

Treating ADHD with NBP
Phase II: Treatment

This phase of treatment deals with the application of dietary supplements and interventions to the treatment of ADHD in a systematic and categorical way. Supplement prescription is discussed in detail along with specific dietary interventions, which, in some cases, may be used adjunctively or in lieu of supplements.

Discuss the Role of Dietary Modifications with Patients and Parents

At some point during the treatment phase, it is important to discuss the beneficial role of dietary modifications. After hearing facts about how dietary changes can help, some patients will want to start implementing them immediately. Others may see such interventions as too extreme, invasive to daily routines, or something to fall back on only if and when supplements and/or medications fail or are only partially effective. In any case, introducing these concepts early and providing specific suggestions for dietary adjustments gives clients the opportunity to begin treatment in an ideal way or to file these ideas away for further use, if necessary.

As it relates to scholastic performance, breakfast is arguably the most important meal of the day and one over which parents probably have the most control. Incorporating the nutrients that address ADHD symptoms early in the day is a great treatment strategy. Keep in mind that dietary approaches must take into account which foods children are likely to eat. Encouraging experimentation and flexibility is key.

Increase Dietary Omega-3 Fats
Omega-3 fats (n-3 fats) are required for life and must be obtained through the diet because our bodies cannot synthesize them.

Alpha-linolenic acid (ALA) is an n-3 fat from plant sources like flax, chia, canola, and hemp. Eicosapentaenoic acid (EPA) and docosahexaenoic acid (DHA) are n-3 fats made by our bodies and derived from animal sources like certain species of cold water fish (salmon, mackerel, herring, sardines, anchovies) and grass-fed and game animals. ALA must be converted to EPA and DHA by our bodies in order to be used directly in the central nervous system.

As we will see, this conversion can be sluggish and low yielding. N-3 fats are metabolized to chemicals called *prostaglandins*, *leukotrienes*, and *thromboxanes*, which have anti-inflammatory, antithrombotic (anticlot), and vasodilatory (relaxes the vascular system) effects. The n-6 fats, found in most vegetable oils like corn, safflower, sunflower, and soy, as well as nuts and avocados, are also considered to be essential. These fats are metabolized to different prostaglandins, leukotrienes, and thromboxanes that are proinflammatory, promote thrombosis, and are vaso-constrictive. A notable exception to this is the anti-inflammatory n-6 fat gamma-linolenic acid (GLA), which is produced in small quantities by the body from linoleic acid and found in some foods[135] and oils, like borage and evening primrose. Simopoulos describes in a 2011 article in *Molecular Neurobiology* how over vast periods of evolutionary time, human diets contained a ratio of n-6 to n-3 fats that was approximately 1:1. N-3 fats were found in all foods that were consumed by humans.[136]

This dietary environment, in turn, exerted influences on genetic selection, which, in conjunction with other environmental factors, governed the development and functioning of all systems of the body. Agribusiness and food technology have drastically changed the nutritional landscape in which we develop and live. An increase in the dietary n-6:n-3 ratio from 1:1 to approximately 15:1 over the past 100 to 150 years, along with decreased levels of antioxidants, helps predispose modern humans to cancers, obesity, arthritis, asthma, and cardiovas-cular inflammatory and autoimmune diseases.[137]

Case Study B

A nine-year-old boy received a diagnosis of ADHD combined type (inattention, hyperactivity, and impulsivity) on the basis of ADHD symptom checklist scores and direct observation. He was treatment naïve. Attempts were made to obtain laboratory tests, but he was resistant due to fear of needles. Family history was significant for ADHD with jitters associated with even low doses of stimulant medications. His parents preferred to avoid the use of prescription medications and stimulants, if possible.

Treatment began with standard recommendations for omega-3 fats, magnesium, and a probiotic, as well as basic information about nutrition. He started with two teaspoons of fish oil in the evening (360mg of EPA and 360mg of DHA). He was unable to take the magnesium because the tablets were too big. His mother was unable to find the recommended probiotic at the store. After taking only the omega-3 fat supplement (which he actually loved the taste of and asked for nightly) for about three weeks, his parents noted that he was somewhat less hyperactive.

We discussed increasing the dose to six teaspoons per night (1080mg of EPA and 1080mg of DHA) and trying a powdered magnesium supplement. Six weeks later, his mother reported that fish oil was having a profound effect on his ADHD symptoms, especially the hyperactivity. Other members of the family also noticed this and commented about it. For the first time in school, he was getting all A's on his work. Because he was doing so well with fish oil only, the parents opted to continue only this intervention. Results have been stable for an additional three to four months thus far.

> This case is an unusual example of how monotherapy with omega-3 fats effectively treated ADHD symptoms after one to two months at an appropriate dose. I must emphasize that this type of robust effect by using only essential fats is not the norm and should not be expected, but it does occur. It would have been interesting to know what his RBC n-6:n-3 ratio was before and after this treatment.

Why Omega-3s Have Decreased in the Food Supply

Although the economic drive to produce food at a lower cost allows us to feed ourselves more efficiently than ever, the nature of the foods produced have essentially changed. Convenience, processed, and packaged foods are commonly laden with large of amounts of n-6 fats, such as corn, sunflower, cottonseed, and other vegetable oils. Moreover, these fats are often converted into *trans fats*, which are primarily novel synthetic compounds produced by the process of hydrogenation,[138] making them solids at room temperature and improving their stability and shelf life. Trans fats decrease the production of n-3 fats via enzyme inhibition and have been associated with aggression and irritability.[139]

Industrialized production of meats and dairy products supplants n-3s with n-6s. It has become the norm for live-stock to be confined to feedlots for eating grains, which are high in n-6 fats, as opposed to grazing and roaming. Grass-fed, forage-fed, or free-range livestock consume higher amounts of n-3s and lower amounts of n-6s and spend more time roaming and foraging for food. Meat from grass- or forage-fed livestock, as opposed to grain-fed livestock, has more n-3s,[140] less satu-rated fat,[141] and more precursors to vitamins A and E, as well as the endogenous antioxidants glutathione and superoxide dismutase. In one study, 30 animals were forage fed, and the n-6:n-3 ratio in the meat was compared with that in standard grain-fed livestock; the n-6:n-3 ratio in forage-fed livestock was 2.6 to 3 as opposed to that in the grain-fed livestock, which was 16.8 to 28.9.[142]

In a double-blind placebo-controlled study, 20 healthy meat eaters were given grass-fed meat three times per day for four weeks, which resulted in significantly increased levels of n-3 fats in their plasma and platelets.[143] Cheese from grass-fed cows has four times the n-3 fats and decreased n-6s when compared with cheese from grain-fed cows.[144] The current industrialized food production methods are prime and pervasive examples of how trying to produce food as inexpensively as possible has direct bearings on our health.

Reasons to Increase Omega-3s
To illustrate the effect of how dietary fats affect our nervous system, consider the analogy of the cell phone. Imagine that a cell phone is like one of the neurons in the brain. It is constantly placing calls to other neurons as well as receiving them. When the fats located in the membrane of the cell are optimal with high levels of n-3s, as well as limited amounts of n-6s and toxic fats (trans fats, heated and oxidized polyunsaturated fats, and saturated fats), it's like having full bars with great reception. Messages are sent and received clearly and consistently. Conversely, when n-6 and trans fat ratios are too high, the signal is impaired.

These cell communication problems may contribute to the presentation and severity of psychiatric symptoms and disorders. Therefore, it is advisable to make dietary choices that maximize "good" fats (n-3s) and minimize "bad" ones (n-6s).

How to Increase Omega-3s
One of the best ways to accomplish this is by choosing wild fish high in n-3 fats and grass- or forage-fed meats and dairy products instead of grain-fed, feedlot-raised animals. It's really not surprising that what animals eat and what we eat (by exten-

sion) influence our biochemistry for better or worse. Although incorporating flax, chia, and hemp seeds, as well as canola oil, into the diet will help to ensure a high intake of plant-based n-3 fats, these must be converted by the body to EPA and DHA for use in the central nervous system.

The other side of the equation is to reduce the intake of n-6 and trans fats by avoiding common polyunsaturated oils found in many packaged and prepared foods, including corn, soy, sunflower, safflower, and other vegetable oils, as well as hydrogenated oils (trans fats).

It is also advisable to avoid cooking with polyunsaturated n-6 and n-3 fats because they are easily oxidized by oxygen and heat to form high levels of toxic lipid peroxides. When oils high in alpha-linolenic acid (ALA), such as canola or flax oil, are heated, they form carcinogens and mutagens (cancer-causing agents).[145] With this in mind, it is generally best to cook with fats that are naturally solid at room temperature, such as virgin coconut oil, ghee (clarified butter), free-range lard, and goose or duck fat (animal tallow) because they remain stable at high temperatures.[146]

Increase omega-3 fats in the diet by:

- choosing meat and dairy products from grass-fed or forage-raised livestock as well as eggs high in omega-3 fats, and

- increasing dietary intake of flax, chia, and hemp seeds (these may be sprinkled on cereals or added to trail mix or smoothies) and canola oil (do not heat or fry because this will denature the fats and defeat the purpose).

Decrease omega-6 fats and toxic fats in the diet by:

- avoiding corn, soy, safflower, sunflower, and other vege-table oils (unheated olive oil is OK);

- avoiding partially hydrogenated fats, vegetable shortening, margarine, and fried foods in general; and

- using fats that are solid at room temperature for cooking, such as coconut oil (choose raw and without any additives) or organic butter or ghee (clarified butter).

Dietary Modifications to Avoid Fluctuations in Blood Sugar

Fluctuations in blood sugar can occur when large amounts of sugar, flour, or other processed carbohydrates are ingested without other nutrients, such as healthy fats, proteins, and/or fiber. When processed carbohydrates are eaten alone, there is nothing to slow down their absorption into the body, and blood sugar rises rapidly. The pancreas then secretes insulin, which quickly reduces the elevated blood sugar but may over-correct, leading to low blood sugar. This, in turn, stimulates a response by the adrenal glands, thereby triggering the production of epinephrine and norepinephrine. At high levels, these hormones can cause hyperactive behaviors.[147] Avoiding rapidly absorbed sucrose-containing foods in young children may prevent diet-related exacerbations of ADHD.[148] Choosing unprocessed foods and eating meals that are balanced in carbohydrates, fats, proteins, and fibers can be effective in this regard.

Diets high in protein and low in carbohydrates (especially sugars) may reduce hyperactivity. When large amounts of unopposed sugars are consumed, such behaviors return.[149] Breakfast, considered the most important meal of the day, is often the least nutritionally balanced meal. For some children, common breakfast foods include processed cereals and breads without sufficient fiber, protein, and healthy fats; these foods can lead to a sugar crash with associated exacerbation of ADHD symptoms and cravings for more of the same types of foods. This situation can create a vicious cycle that compromises mental and physical functioning in those with and those without ADHD.

Recommendations Include:
Avoiding sugar, flour, and other high-carbohydrate processed foods (soda, bread, pasta, rice cakes, popcorn, crackers, etc.) in general. Choose breads that are "flourless" (those made with sprouted grains). When such foods are eaten, make sure they are consumed with other foods that will slow down the absorption process—such as healthy fats (raw nuts, nut butters, seeds, coconut oil, whole milk from grass-fed livestock, or cheeses, etc.), proteins (meats from grass-fed or forage-raised livestock, eggs, cheese, fish), and/or fiber (raw nuts, seeds, fruits, and vegetables). Raw or dried fruit is acceptable in moderation, as it contains fiber and important healthy phytochemicals.

Smoothies for breakfast or anytime: combine ingredients, such as milk, coconut water, fruit juice, fruit, flax, chia or hemp seeds, and protein powder in a blender for a delicious and well-balanced breakfast or snack that will give you a steady supply of energy for mental and physical tasks without leading to a sugar crash.

Suggested Protein Supplements Include:
Mt. Capra goat milk protein: caprotein and whey protein products

Sunwarrior vegetarian protein powders: raw, sprouted, whole-grain brown rice protein or Warrior Blend

Whey protein from grass-fed cows

Suggested flax supplements include organic sprouted flax seeds from Organic Traditions and Sprout Revolution

Avoid Pesticides

Organophosphates are common pesticides used in the United States. According to the National Academy of Sciences, the major source of exposure for infants and children is in their diets.[150] The developing brain is more susceptible to the negative effects of neurotoxins in pesticides, so children are at highest risk for adverse effects.[151] Six- to 11-year-old children have the highest levels of urinary dialkyl phosphate (a pesticide) metabolites of any age group in the US population.[152] This may be at least partly because children have decreased expression of enzymes that metabolize pesticides.[153]

Risks of Pesticide Exposure

Prenatal exposure to pesticides is associated with increased risk of pervasive developmental disorder and delays in mental development at two and three years of age.[154] Childhood pesticide exposure is associated with behavioral problems, decreased performance in short-term memory and motor skills, and longer reaction times.[155] Data from several studies have linked ADHD symptom presence and severity with exposure to pesticides.[156] The evidence is clear that pesticides from food have adverse effects on the developing nervous system and in some cases may be exacerbating and even causing ADHD and other developmental problems.

How do we avoid pesticide ingestion? Choosing organic foods is the best way to ensure that what we eat is pesticide free. However, this can be an expensive proposition and one that may be difficult to carry out. Incorporate organic foods that children are likely to eat as much as possible. To whatever degree we can strive for this, we protect our children's vulnerable nervous systems as well as our own.

Some Recommendations for Parents and Patients:

Try to buy and eat as much organic food as possible. Work slowly toward increasing the amount over time. Some nonorganic foods are safer than others in terms of pesticide residues. These tend to be food with peels or skins that are not consumed or are not significantly threatened by insect pests and therefore require few or no pesticides. Such foods include avocado, bananas, pineapple, kiwi, mango, papaya, asparagus, broccoli, and onions.

For other foods, we should try to buy organic whenever possible. These include most soft fruits with thin and edible skin, berries, lettuces, leafy greens, bell peppers, potatoes, carrots, cucumbers, cauliflower, and tomatoes. The Environmental Working Group puts out an annual list of the foods with the most and least pesticides at https://www.ewg.org/foodnews/index.php. They estimate that individuals can reduce their exposure to pesticides by 80% if they just avoid certain foods that are nonorganic.

The following is a list of companies making snacks and bars that are organic, often raw, and taste great, so kids are more likely to eat them: Go Raw products, Raw Revolution Bars, Lydia's products, Pure Bars, Organic Food Bar products, SHANTI bars, Marigold bars, Donnabar organic bars, and Raw Crunch Bars. Having such snacks available provides a convenient alternative to snacks that are high in sugar and low in fiber and may have pesticide residues or artificial additives.

Restrictive and Elimination Diets

Adverse reactions to food or food components, including artificial food colorings, flavorings, and preservatives, may be associated with behavioral disturbances in ADHD.[157] When ADHD symptoms develop in response to food components and immunological mechanisms can be identified, then ADHD symptoms may, in part, be due to an allergic response.[158] Differences in genes that regulate histamine metabolism in clients with ADHD are one likely connection between food allergies and ADHD symptoms.[159] As a contributing factor to ADHD symptoms, a true allergy to foods is best determined by improvement during an elimination diet followed by an exacerbation of symptoms when the offending agent is reintroduced.[160]

A restrictive or elimination diet aims to remove the most common allergens from the diet that may cause or exacerbate symptoms of ADHD. Multiple studies have examined the effect of such diets on core symptoms. One of the limiting factors of such research is the varied definition of a restricted diet:

The most commonly studied diets all eliminate artificial food colorings and flavorings in addition to other foods.

The Feingold diet also removes preservatives and artificial sweeteners.

The oligoantigenic diet only allows for specific foods: banana, apple, pear, cruciferous vegetables, lamb, chicken, and water.

The "few foods" diet only allows for lamb, turkey, rice, vegetables, fruits, tea, pears, vegetable oil, and water.

Other restrictive diets eliminate dairy, wheat and gluten, corn, sugar, chocolate, and caffeine.

Open-label trials of such diets do produce reliable and clinically significant benefits for children with ADHD at a response rate of about 33%.[161] Although caution must be used when interpreting the significance and applicability of data from open-label trials, these reported results should be considered when making clinical decisions and recommendations: One-third of all children with ADHD had clinically significant improvement when such diets were implemented.

When synthetic food additives were studied, event rates (exacerbation of ADHD symptoms when food additives were ingested) were found in approximately 8% of all children with ADHD. Artificial food colorings (AFCs) have not been found to be causative in ADHD, but there may be a subgroup of patients who do show significant improvement when they are eliminated from the diet and exacerbation of symptoms when they are reintroduced.[162,163,164,165,166] In a meta-analysis of double-blind placebo-controlled (DBPC) trials examining the effects of AFC on ADHD symptoms,[167] the effect size was approximately one-third to one-half of the effect size calculated in a meta-analysis of trials evaluating methylphenidate as a treatment for ADHD. When artificial food colorings were added back into the diet, this was about one-third to one-half of the effect of taking children off stimulant medications. Ironically, all classes of prescription medications indicated for the treatment of ADHD (stimulants, atomoxetine, and alpha-2 agonists) frequently contain AFCs.

Given these findings, why are restrictive and elimination diets implemented so infrequently? Constant bombardment with advertising for convenience, novelty, and fast foods from an early age; the availability of such foods outside the home; social pressures to eat as peers do; and the changes that are required of the family system as a whole—coupled with the ease, convenience, and marketing that accompany stimulant and other medications (which have a much higher response rate but miss important nutritional factors)—largely relegate elimination diets to a last resort.

Case Study C

A man in his early 20s with a diagnosis of ADHD inattentive subtype, as well as anxiety, responded quite well to prescription stimulant medication and an SSRI along with psychotherapy. Although the symptoms of these diagnoses were much improved to a near subclinical level, he reported a feeling of mental sluggishness and fogginess occurring after nearly every meal. These symptoms were so problematic that he began skipping breakfast and lunch, for the most part, and only eating later in the day when mental acuity was not as important.

He noted that when eating later in the day, he experienced symptoms consistent with an allergic response along with the mental sluggishness. Commonly, the allergic

---

symptoms would make it difficult for him to initiate and maintain sleep. After some discussion, he had food-allergy testing performed and found that he had sensitivities to dairy products, wheat (gluten), eggs, and several other foods. After examining his diet, he realized that he had been consuming one or more of these foods at virtually every meal. After eliminating the offending foods, he was able to eat during the day without adverse effects, his sleep improved, and significantly better control of his ADHD symptoms was achieved. He commented that although he had to give up many of the foods he enjoyed, eliminating them had a profound effect on his life and sense of well-being.

This case underscores the improvement in symptom control and quality of life possible when allergic and hypersensitivity components of the diet are effectively addressed.

How to Implement Restrictive or Elimination Diets

Using such approaches is not as painful or impossible as it may seem. What is required is a period of diligence and patience while determining which foods or food components are causing problems. Once identified, these foods can be eliminated from the diet as much as possible. This can be achieved by implementing a highly restrictive diet for several weeks and assessing whether the patient has derived significant benefit. Then, introduce foods back into the diet one at a time, for a period of one to two weeks per food, while carefully monitoring maintenance of improvement versus exacerbation of symptoms. The result of this process is arriving at the least-restrictive diet that minimizes the adverse effect of food reactions.

Alternatively, it's possible to start with the current diet and systematically remove only one type of food or additive at a time. This approach requires less adjustment but takes a longer time to get results. In either case, the effects on attention, hyperactivity, and impulsivity symptoms achievable by dietary manipulation alone can be significant.

Treating Nonbreathing-Related Sleep Disturbances

Sleep disorders not related to allergic rhinitis or breathing-related difficulties should be addressed prior to or in conjunction with treatment with essential nutrients (see the next section). Evidence suggests that the following interventions have specific efficacy for sleep-related problems in the setting of ADHD.

L-Theanine

L-Theanine at a glance:

May address: Improves sleep parameters in the setting of ADHD

Dose: 200-500mg 1 hour prior to bedtime

Time to onset of action: 30-60 minutes

Adverse events (AEs): Rarely sedation at high doses

GRAS: Yes

L-Theanine (not to be confused with the B vitamin thiamine or the amino acid L-threonine) occurs naturally in tea leaves and may improve sleep efficiency (time spent in restful sleep) and sleep activity (decrease bouts of nocturnal activity). This is one of the best-tolerated supplements used in clinical practice, with the rarely occurring side effect of sedation at higher doses. Of note, it blunts the excitatory effects of caffeine.[168] Therefore, when taken during the day, patients who need their morning cup(s) of coffee should be advised to drink it before taking L-theanine.

L-Theanine has GRAS status granted by the FDA in 2006 and is intended as a food additive with a mean estimated intake of 628mg per day; it tends to be stimulating at low doses and sedating at high doses.[169] It is not considered mutagenic, carcinogenic, or genotoxic in animals or bacteria.[170] L-Theanine and its metabolites reach peak concentrations in plasma within a few hours and rapidly decrease via urinary excretion. It is no longer found in plasma or brain tissue 24 hours after oral administration and, therefore, is not likely to accumulate in the body.[171] Human studies regarding safety, tolerability, pregnancy, nursing, and fertility are lacking; however, inferences may be made based on long-term observational data on tea drinkers and consumption of L-theanine as a dietary supplement.

Evidence for the Efficacy of L-Theanine in Treating Sleep Disorders Associated with ADHD
A randomized controlled study in 98 boys with DSM-IV ADHD given L-theanine 200mg twice a day (morning and afternoon) for six weeks resulted in improvements in sleep efficiency (increased time in restful sleep) as measured by means of actigraphy ($p<0.05$) and sleep activity (decreased bouts of nocturnal activity; $p<0.05$).[172] No significant differences were found for sleep latency or duration.

Suggested Use:
Although the evidence indicates that 200mg twice a day (morning and afternoon) is effective, taking it at bedtime seems to give better results. Start with 200mg approximately one hour prior to bedtime. This may be titrated nightly up to 500mg or more. In general, however, if no improvements in sleep are seen by 300 to 400mg, it is unlikely to be effective at higher doses.

Suntheanine® is a form of L-theanine that many manufacturers use in products widely available in 100 and 200mg capsules. Often, other purported sleep-promoting and stress-relieving substances will be included with L-theanine, so read labels carefully.

Case Study D

A 12-year-old boy with a family history of bipolar and depressive disorders was diagnosed with ADHD inattentive subtype when he was eight years old. In fourth grade, he was prescribed methylphenidate, which improved ADHD symptoms but caused significant irritability in the afternoon when the medication wore off. He was switched to a long-acting form of dexmethylphenidate, which had a therapeutic effect but had negative effects on the spontaneity of his personality, sense of humor, and, as a result, social interaction. This is a commonly observed side effect of stimulant medications. Later, he developed a neck tic and an ocular tic (blinking). The psychiatrist at the time tried to address these with guanfacine, a medication frequently prescribed for ADHD. However, after taking it for one day, the client became emotionally distraught, tearful, and jumpy. He experienced sensitivity to light and sound. These adverse effects dissipated when the medication was discontinued.

The client was next tried on a long-acting form of methylphenidate, but it caused insomnia, even at a low dose, so he was switched back to dexmethylphenidate at a lower dose, which obviated the majority of adverse effects (tics and personality changes) but did not fully address his ADHD symptoms. In sixth grade, he was tried on lisdexamfetamine, a time-release form of dextroamphetamine, and the dose was titrated to 25mg. The low dose of this medication did not affect his personality as other stimulants did, according to the client, family, and teachers, while affording moderate control of his ADHD symptoms.

Prior to my evaluation, he had also been briefly tried on amphetamine salts, but within 45 minutes, he complained of nausea and exhaustion, and within two hours, he was tearful and upset.

Upon presentation for evaluation, he had been taking 27mg of lisdexamfetamine for several months with moderate control of ADHD symptoms, early insomnia about 25% of the time, and some decrease in appetite. He was in a pattern of taking the medication only on school days with weekends and holidays off, which mitigated effects on sleep and appetite. Laboratory test results revealed normal levels of ferritin, zinc, and vitamin D.

The client was started on a multivitamin and appropriate doses of omega-3 fats, magnesium, and a probiotic. The client's mother had read about an amino acid called *glycine*, which has evidence-based sleep-promoting effects,[173,174,175] although not necessarily in the context of ADHD. The time it took him to fall asleep (sleep latency) reduced markedly; however, he experienced daytime sedation. The glycine was titrated down from 1000 to 500mg and was eventually discontinued, which eliminated the daytime sedation but increased sleep latency. L-Theanine 300mg at bedtime was added, and it worked quite well for insomnia without sedation the next day. Most mornings he also had a smoothie for breakfast that included a high level of protein.

After approximately one month on the following regimen, the client and parents reported significantly improved focus and sleep:

Protein-rich smoothie in the morning

Lisdexamfetamine: 27mg in the morning

One multivitamin in the morning

Omega-3 fats: 1500mg of EPA per day

Ultra Jarro-Dophilus: one capsule per day

Magnesium citrate: 320mg at bedtime

L-Theanine: 300mg at bedtime and 200mg in the morning

His mother was interested in what could be done to decrease or eliminate the use of the prescription medication. We added acetyl-L-carnitine (ALCAR) and titrated the dose to 300mg in the morning and again in the early afternoon. This seemed to potentiate the effect of the stimulant, and we tried him without the medication for several days at the end of the semester and during Christmas break. Prior to break, his teachers remarked that his class participation improved and that he seemed more spontaneous and comfortable with a larger variety of students. However, he would sometimes lose focus, get off track, and need more redirection. His parents noticed that he would giggle more, act silly, and be somewhat hyperactive. As the break ensued, concern grew that he was too giddy and ungrounded.

He returned to school on ALCAR 500mg in the morning and 250mg in the early afternoon, along with lisdexamfetamine 15mg. It was apparent that the ALCAR was moving him towards hypomania. Given the family history of bipolarity and the known side effects of ALCAR, this supplement was discontinued. Next, we tried phosphatidylserine (PS) and titrated the dose up to 300mg in the morning and 200mg in the early afternoon, while decreasing the lisdexamfetamine to 20mg. After four to five weeks, this resulted in the client becoming more mindful and taking his time on homework and tests. Rushing through school work had previously been a problem. This combination was effective for some time, with some mild to moderate complaints of affective blunting and decreased sense of humor.

In an effort to reduce the dose of stimulant medication further, we tried N-acetylcysteine (NAC) and titrated up to 1200mg twice per day without any discernible effects. After discontinuing NAC, we added pycnogenol at 50mg in the morning and early afternoon. This seemed to improve his ability to do homework into the late afternoon, but did not allow us to decrease the dose of the stimulant lower than 20mg.

As he entered high school, he began to complain about excessive sweating on the days he took lisdexamfetamine, so we discussed alternative medications. After some discussion, we decided to try a medication called *bupropion*, which is an antidepressant used off-label for ADHD. Other members of the family had used this medication at low to moderate doses with good effect. Once the switch was made, the sweating remitted, and he felt more socially outgoing and spontaneous with good control of ADHD symptoms. The dose of bupropion was titrated to 75mg in the morning and 75mg in the early afternoon.

His current regimen includes the following:

Protein-rich smoothie in the morning

One multivitamin in the morning

Bupropion: 75mg in the morning and afternoon

PS: 300mg in the morning and 200mg in the afternoon

Pycnogenol: 50mg in the morning and 50mg in the afternoon

Omega-3 fats: 1500mg of EPA per day

Ultra Jarro-Dophilus: one capsule per day

Magnesium citrate: 320mg at bedtime

L-Theanine: 300mg at bedtime and 200mg in the morning alternating with melatonin 1 to 3mg at bedtime

This case highlights the following:

Stimulant medications address symptoms of ADHD effectively but with the common adverse events of decreased appetite, insomnia, and lack of spontaneity and humor or being overly serious, which necessitated a decreased dose leading to breakthrough symptoms.

The use of NBP allowed for a decreased dose of medication but, in this case, did not adequately control ADHD symptoms without the adjunctive use of medication.

A client with a family history of bipolar disorder developed symptoms consistent with hypomania when taking ALCAR. L-Theanine provided effective control of insomnia associated with stimulant medication.

The family and client were willing to adhere to a complex medication, supplement, and dietary regimen.

Melatonin

Melatonin at a glance:

May address: Sleep parameters in the setting of ADHD; mitigates adverse effects of stimulant medication on sleep

Dose: 1-6mg at bedtime

Time to onset of action: 30-60 minutes

AEs: See full details in text

GRAS: No

Possible MOA: Possibly GABAergic

Melatonin is a hormone produced from the amino acid tryptophan by the pineal gland in response to darkness, establishing a daily circadian rhythm. The most common adverse events are nausea, headache, and dizziness, but these are not significantly different from placebo and do not change with dose.[176] Associated nightmares and hypotension are rare and mild.[177] Very high doses can cause cognitive and motor impairment, as well as decreased body temperature.[178]

Since 1993, it has been classified as an orphan medication for the treatment of circadian rhythm sleep disorders in blind patients without any light perception, and it is currently not FDA approved.[179] The half-life is short (33-47 minutes)[180]; therefore, it is not likely to accumulate in the body over time.

It crosses the blood-brain barrier and is metabolized by the cytochrome P450 enzyme CYP1A2.[181] Exogenous melatonin is relatively safe even at high doses; it tends to be nontoxic, and an LD50 (or the dose required to kill 50% of a population of test animals) could not be obtained even at extremely high doses.[182] In humans, 6g per day for one month led to no major adverse events except gastrointestinal upset and residual sleepiness.[183]

Exogenous melatonin is currently contraindicated during pregnancy and breast-feeding, as safety data in humans is lacking.[184] Theoretically, it may interfere with development during puberty, but this has not been observed clinically.[185] Studies on melatonin at 2mg per day for up to one year show no tolerance, no rebound insomnia, no withdrawal symptoms, and no suppression of endogenous production.[186]

Melatonin may potentiate the effects of anticoagulants and increase the risk of bleeding.[187] In normotensive subjects receiving 5mg of melatonin daily over 4 weeks, both systolic and diastolic blood pressure decreased significantly ($p < 0.05$).[188] Use caution when administering melatonin with antihypertensives like clonidine.[189] Melatonin may have immunostimulant or immunosuppressant activity depending upon the state of the immune system. As such, it could interfere with the efficacy of immunosuppressant medications.

Melatonin generally acts as a potent anti-inflammatory. However, in certain clinical situations like rheumatoid arthritis and asthma,[190] it may have inflammatory effects.[191] In some cases (juvenile intractable epilepsy), melatonin acts as an anticonvulsant,[192] and in other clinical settings (such as temporal lobe epilepsy and neurological disabilities in children), it appears to induce electroencephalographic abnormalities and increase the incidence of seizures.[193]

Melatonin may potentiate the effects of GABA (gamma-aminobutyric acid, an inhibitory neurotransmitter) and GABAergic medications, as well as other sedatives, so use with caution.[194] Melatonin should be used with caution or may be relatively contraindicated in patients taking antidepressants, birth control pills, blood pressure medications, anticoagulants and immunosuppressants.[195]

Evidence for the Efficacy of Melatonin in Treating Sleep Disorders Associated with ADHD

In a DBPC study, 105 medication-free six- to 12-year-olds with ADHD and chronic early insomnia were given melatonin 3 or 6mg for four weeks.[196] Actigraphy showed advanced sleep onset ($p < 0.001$), increased total sleep time ($p < 0.01$), increased sleep efficiency ($p < 0.01$), and decreased nocturnal restlessness ($p < 0.03$). Additionally, sleep logs showed decreased difficulty falling asleep ($p < 0.0001$). However, there were no significant effects on problem behaviors, cognitive performance, or quality of life.

In another DBPC study, 50 children with ADHD combined type from the ages of seven to 12 were given 3 or 6mg of melatonin (weight based) or placebo along with methylphenidate 1mg per kilogram of body weight per day for eight weeks.[197] The melatonin group exhibited significantly decreased sleep latency scores (23.15±15.25 versus 17.96±11.66) and total sleep disturbance scores (48.84±13.42 versus 41.30±9.67) before and after melatonin administration. Total sleep time improvement in the melatonin group nearly reached significance ($p < 0.06$). The authors concluded that melatonin given along with methylphenidate in children with ADHD may improve height, weight, growth, and development because of improved sleep parameters and possibly increased growth hormone release during sleep.

Suggested Use:
Start with 1mg taken one hour prior to bedtime and titrate nightly by 1mg to a maximum of 6mg. Melatonin at 3 to 6mg every night at bedtime is likely safe and effective for ADHD-related sleep problems, including increased sleep latency, decreased total sleep time, decreased sleep efficiency, and increased nocturnal restlessness. Melatonin may have a role in the adjunctive application of NBP by mitigating potential adverse effects of stimulant medications on sleep parameters.

Melatonin is widely available from a number of manufacturers. Immediate-release formulas are quite effective for sleep latency issues but may result in awakening several hours into sleep. In such cases, time-release melatonin is suggested or a combination of immediate- and time-release melatonin.

Magnesium
Magnesium at a glance:

May address: Sleep difficulties in a number of settings (not ADHD specifically)

Dose: 6-9mg/kg at bedtime

Time to onset of action: 30-60 minutes

AEs: Sedation and loose stools, also see full *Physicians' Desk Reference* entry

GRAS: Yes

Possible MOA: Neurotransmitter synthesis, GABAergic, serotonergic

Magnesium is an essential mineral that has myriad functions in the human body.

Evidence for the Efficacy of Magnesium in Treating Sleep Disorders Associated with ADHD

There are no specific studies examining the relationship between ADHD-associated sleep difficulties and magnesium. However, research indicates that magnesium may be effective for age-related sleep changes,[198] alcohol-related sleep dysfunction,[199] and chronic stress and sleep deprivation.[200]

Suggested Use:

Anecdotally, magnesium citrate, Mg glycinate, Mg taurate, or Mg threonate weight-based dosing at 6-9mg/kg at bedtime may be effective for sleep problems associated with ADHD. Please see the section under "Essential Nutrients" in the following chapter for full prescribing suggestions.

Chapter 11

Prescribing Nutritional Supplements for ADHD

Supplements used for the treatment of ADHD can be divided into three major categories: essential, metabolic, and herbal. In general, the essential and metabolic categories of supplements have GRAS status and come in prescription versions with uses recognized by mainstream medicine.

Although herbs often have long histories of human consumption and evidence for medicinal use is increasing, they are not essential for life and most of them do not have GRAS status. Additionally, relatively less is known about the pharmacodynamics, safety, toxicity, and long-term use of many herbs. Although there is some compelling evidence that certain herbs may be useful in addressing ADHD symptoms, many also have hormonal and endocrine effects, which could conservatively render them contraindicated in children and adolescents unless certain laboratory test values are monitored. Therefore, it is prudent to start with the essential, then metabolic nutritional interventions, and finally try certain herbs in a time-limited way, if necessary.

Prescribing Essential Nutrients

The essential nutrients used in NBP to treat ADHD include essential fatty acids, magnesium, vitamin B6, zinc, iron, vitamin D3, a multivitamin/mineral, and probiotics. Ideally, by the time the treatment phase begins, laboratory test values are available, including RBC n-6:n-3 ratio, RBC Mg, serum zinc, ferritin, and vitamin D. In some cases, however, RBC n-6:n-3 ratios and RBC Mg may be cost prohibitive. When levels of these nutrients are low or out of balance (in the case of n-3 fats), supplementation addresses the associated deficiencies.

These interventions may improve the synthesis and metabolism of important neurotransmitters by providing required cofactors for enzymatic reactions and address oxidative stress. Given the risk-to-benefit ratio for these essential nutrients, treating empirically with a multinutrient approach as supported by research is advised. Therefore, when implementing a comprehensive NBP approach, the following essential nutrients are prescribed concurrently for a period of several weeks up to two months prior to prescribing metabolic and herbal nutrients, if necessary. Concurrent administration is achieved by adding supplements to the regimen one at a time with approximately three to five days between each. Implementation in a stepwise fashion helps to pinpoint supplements that may be causing adverse effects.

Omega-3 Fats
Omega-3 fats at a glance:

May address: Inattention, hyperactivity, oppositionality, aggression

Dose: 1000-5000mg EPA daily

Time to onset: 2-4 weeks

AEs: Gastrointestinal upset, fishy aftertaste (see full details in text)

GRAS: Yes

Prescription forms: Yes

Possible MOA: IIO axis, membrane-lipid therapy, dopaminergic, serotonergic

Evidence for the Efficacy of Omega-3 Fats in Treating ADHD
Throughout anyone's lifetime, a sufficient supply of essential fatty acids is necessary for healthy functioning. This is particularly true for the nervous system, which includes the brain. Neurologic development occurs rapidly during gestation and the postnatal period. Fetuses and infants are particularly

sensitive to a lack of these critical nutrients. Evidence in the literature strongly suggests that deficiencies of essential fatty acids during development lead to dysfunctions of the nervous system, including visual, psychomotor, and cognitive deficits, whereas supplementation improves neurologic functioning.[201] The majority of observational studies investigating various n-3 and n-6 fatty acid levels and ADHD symptoms have found significant correlations between lower n-3 and higher omega-6 levels and ADHD symptom presence and severity in children and adults.[202]

This is also the case for dyslexia, dyspraxia, and other learning disabilities.[203] A subset of children with ADHD and other learning disabilities may have deficiencies of n-3 fats along with an increased nutritional requirement for them. A study that examined serum levels of EPA and DHA in 29 boys with ADHD compared with levels in 43 boys without the diagnosis found that callous/unemotional traits were significantly and nega-tively related to both EPA and the total omega-3 levels in the ADHD group.[204]

Tissue availability of essential fatty acids depends both on dietary intake and metabolic turnover.[205] The conversion of ALA (vegetable derived n-3 fats) to EPA and DHA is a slow and low-yield process. It is estimated to take approximately 20g of pure ALA to make just 1g of EPA.[206] This conversion process can be affected by genetic, hormonal, and nutritional factors. Fatty acid desaturase gene clusters 1 and 2 (FADS1 and FADS2) code for enzymes that are crucial in the metabolism of essential fatty acids, particularly with regard to forming the longer chain poly-unsaturated fats like EPA and DHA.

There are close associations between genetic variations in these gene clusters and serum phospholipid contents of essential fatty acids. Fatty acid composition of serum phospholipids is, in part, genetically determined by these clusters. On the basis of gene variation, individuals may require different amounts of essential fatty acids to achieve a similar biologic effect.[207] A significant association has been found between children with ADHD and genetic differences in the FADS2 gene, which codes for the enzyme delta-6 desaturase, the rate-limiting step in the conversion of ALA to EPA and DHA.[208] Hormonal factors may play a significant role in levels of essential fatty acids in the body. Testosterone inhibits the synthesis of long-chain fatty acids like EPA and DHA, whereas estrogen protects them from breakdown.

This may help account for the greater incidence of ADHD and other developmental and learning disabilities in males as opposed to females.[209] The conversion of ALA to longer chain fats requires the mineral factors magnesium and zinc. Deficiencies of these essential nutrients may adversely affect fatty acid profile and neurologic functioning.[210] Conversion is also inhibited by excessive amounts of n-6 fats, which compete with n-3 fats for a limited amount of enzyme activity,[211] as well as the presence of trans fats (hydrogenated oils), which decrease activity of the enzyme delta-6 desaturase.[212] Additionally, children with ADHD may have an increased oxidative breakdown of omega-3 fats. Ethane, a marker of increased oxidation of n-3 fats, was found to be significantly elevated in the breath of children with ADHD when compared with controls.[213] Levels of n-3 fats in our diets and, by extension, in our cells may have a direct effect on levels of dopamine, a neurotransmitter central to the pathophysiology of ADHD.

Rats fed a diet high in n-3 and low in n-6 fats had increased levels of endogenous dopamine in the frontal cortex, a finding thought to be related to decreased activity of monoamine oxidase (MAO)-B (an enzyme that deactivates dopamine).[214] The link between n-3 levels and MAO-B activity could be the phospholipid phosphatidylserine (PS),[215] a component of cellular lipid membranes and a supplement with efficacy in treating ADHD symptoms. A diet low in n-3 fats resulted in decreased levels of PS, which is a selective inhibitor of MAO-B.[216] It follows that decreased PS results in increased MAO-B activity and subsequent decreased levels of dopamine. There is a relatively large body of data on the treatment of ADHD symptoms with n-3 fats. The vast majority of it has been summarized in a systematic review and meta-analysis in the *Journal of the American Academy of Child and Adolescent Psychiatry* published October 2011.[217] Trials that met criteria from 1965 through December 2010 were included and consisted of 10 randomized placebo-controlled trials with a total of 699 participants. The dosages ranged from 250 to 1000mg per day of n-3 fats. Findings indicate a significant effect for overall symptoms (p<0.0001), inattentive symptoms (p<0.009), and hyperactivity (p<0.005). Higher doses of EPA in particular were associated with increased efficacy (p<0.04). Supplementing DHA or ALA was not associated with clinical efficacy.

A length of treatment time ranging from four weeks to four months did not confer greater efficacy over time. Additionally, there were no significant differences between using n-3 fats as monotherapy (using them as the sole intervention) versus using them as augmentation (adding them to other interventions). On the basis of these findings, EPA appears to be the effective n-3 in treating ADHD. High doses may be necessary to achieve a clinical benefit in some cases. Maximal efficacy appears to be achieved within four weeks of initiating treatment.

A meta-regression analysis of randomized controlled trials in children with ADHD receiving polyunsaturated fatty acids was published in 2014; the authors found that the pooled estimate from 18 studies showed that, although combined ADHD symptoms rated by all raters decreased with supplementation to a small but significant degree (p<0.001), this finding was mediated by parent ratings as opposed to teacher ratings.[218] This is a finding that has been observed in previous research. Parents may be better at detecting subtle behavioral changes in their children than teachers are. Interestingly, evidence was strong that the anti-inflammatory n-6 essential fatty acid, gamma-linolenic acid (GLA), and the interaction between GLA and EPA were associated with significant decreases in inattention. A further subgroup analysis confirmed this finding (p<0.0001). Doses of GLA in the six studies that examined combinations of EPA and GLA ranged from 18 to 96mg.

Examining other studies gives additional valuable information affecting clinical decision making. A 12-month randomized controlled trial in 53 six- to 13-year-olds with ADHD, who were given EPA 1109 and DHA 108mg, DHA 1032 and EPA 264mg, or safflower oil containing 1467mg of linoleic acid for four months, found significant associations between increasing levels of RBC EPA and DHA and improved spelling (p<0.001) and attention (p<0.001) and decreased oppositional behaviors (p<0.003), hyperactivity (p<0.001), and cognitive problems (p<0.001).[219] A case-control open-label study with 31 children with ADHD according to DSM-IV criteria evaluated the effects of 210mg per kilogram of body weight per day of EPA and DHA (ratio EPA:DHA = 1.89).[220] For a 40kg child, this would be a total n-3 dose of 8400mg (8.4g) and an EPA dose of about 5.5g. This is a relatively large dose of n-3 fats. At baseline, participants with ADHD had a higher ratio of arachidonic acid (an n-6 fat) to EPA. Over the eight weeks, this ratio significantly decreased from 41.1 to 4.1 (p<0.001). The supplemented group had significantly decreased inattention (p<0.002) and hyperactivity (p<0.007) scores on the parent and teacher Conners' Parent Rating Scale (CPRS) short form. It should be noted that this study had a relatively high number of dropouts for various reasons, including gastrointestinal (GI) upset, refusal to take fish oil, increasing pimples, and the expense of the n-3 fats (apparently, the participants had to pay for it themselves).

In another small, open-label study using very high doses of EPA, nine children with DSM-IV ADHD receiving 10.8g EPA and 5.4g DHA per day for eight weeks had a 71% decrease in their AA:EPA ratio (p<0.01) and showed significant improvement in all categories of the ADHD symptoms checklist (p<0.01-0.05) and on all four categories of the CPRS (p<0.05).[221] Moreover, there was a positive correlation between the percentage change in the AA:EPA ratio and percentage change in severity of illness (p<0.027) but not on other scales.

An additional study using a lower dose of EPA per day gives information about subtypes of children with ADHD that may benefit from n-3 therapy. This was a randomized controlled trial in 92 children with ADHD given only 500mg EPA and 270mg DHA per day for 15 weeks.[222] On the Conners' Teacher Rating Scale (CTRS) there was significant improvement on the inattentive/cognitive subscale only (p<0.04) but not on the total score. When the children with significant oppositional symptoms (n=48) were examined separately, there was improvement on the CTRS total score (p<0.01) and an even greater improvement on the oppositional and inattentive subscales (p<0.001). Children considered to be responders had significantly lower EPA levels (p<0.02) and higher AA:EPA (p<0.05) and AA:DHA (p<0.03) ratios in their serum at baseline.

How to Prescribe Omega-3 Fats for ADHD:
Start with a target dose of approximately 1000 to 1500mg of EPA per day in the form of a high-potency softgel or liquid. Higher doses of 5000 to 10000mg (5-10g) per day may be required for a clinical response in some cases. Evidence suggests that n-3 fats may be effective in treating the core symptoms of ADHD, including inattention and hyperactivity, with clinical improvements starting around two to three weeks and maximizing at approximately four weeks.[223]

A targeted NBP approach could involve prescribing n-3s to address inattention and oppositional symptoms because they may respond preferentially. Along with EPA, most products include a smaller amount of DHA, which co-occurs naturally. Read labels carefully, as often nutritional information on the label is based on two softgels instead of one. Large softgels are difficult for children (and sometimes adults) to swallow.

Alternately, there are several brands of mini-softgels, which are much easier to swallow, but a high number of the softgels are necessary to achieve a therapeutic dose. High-potency liquids are also available from a number of suppliers; they usually come in lemon or orange flavor. Clients tend to prefer them when they are kept at very cold temperatures, as this decreases the flavor.

The most common adverse effects seen clinically are fishy after-taste or fish burps and GI upset. These effects may be decreased or eliminated by using enteric-coated fish oil, taking them just *before* large meals, and/or keeping them in the freezer. It is also a good idea to keep fish oil refrigerated and check manufacturer and expiration dates because EPA, DHA, and polyunsaturated fats, in general, are prone to oxidation due to the increased density of electrons located around double bonds, which may be abducted by free radicals. This oxidation changes the physical and chemical properties of the fats, which alters the cellular membrane adversely. Emphasize to patients that it is important to supplement with EPA as opposed to getting n-3s in the form of ALA from flax or other vegetarian sources because the conversion of ALA to EPA and DHA is a slow and low-yield process.

For clients who are vegetarian or vegan, although there are several brands of nonfish-sourced EPA and DHA supplements, their ratios of EPA to DHA are not ideal for treating ADHD. In order to achieve a more favorable omega-6 to omega-3 ratio, suggest substituting unrefined canola, olive, or coconut oils for corn, soy, safflower, etc.

Substituting meat and dairy from grass- and forage-fed livestock for grain-fed types can also make a significant difference in this regard. In cases of excessively high dietary n-6 intake, these steps may be as important as increasing n-3. The majority of research suggests that n-3 fats act as powerful antioxidants, although there is some evidence they may also act as pro-oxidants. Systematic reviews indicate that n-3s are anti-inflamma-tory[224]; improve markers of cardiovascular risk[225]; and may play preventive or therapeutic roles in type 2 diabetes,[226] nonalco-holic fatty liver disease,[227] metabolic syndrome, obesity,[228] and rheumatoid arthritis.[229]

With regard to psychiatric disorders, the role of n-3 fats is yet to be determined. Numerous studies point to associations between deficiencies and psychological disease, but supple-mentation often produces mixed results. Deficits of n-3 fats are directly related to the prevalence and severity of depression. Putative antidepressant effects of n-3 fats may be mediated by increased serotonergic neurotransmission.[230]

However, a recent systematic review concluded that the effects of supplemental n-3s in depression were not statistically signif-icant.[231] A review of n-3 fats for bipolar disorder indicated that they may be more effective for depressive as opposed to manic symptoms.[232] For autism, only uncontrolled studies have reported a benefit to supplemental n-3 fats.[233] Litera-ture reviews suggest that although DHA and other long-chain fatty acids are decreased in schizophrenia,[234] EPA supplemen-tation is not helpful as an adjunctive treatment in established cases.[235] However, n-3 fats may play a role in prevention in the early stages of psychosis[236] and may address metabolic and extrapyramidal symptoms associated with the use of antipsy-chotic medications.[237] Core symptoms of borderline person-ality disorder,[238] dyslexia,[239] aggression, and impulsivity[240] have responded favorably to supplemental n-3 fats. Elevated n-6:n-3 ratios are associated with cognitive decline and the incidence of dementia.[241] Additional well-controlled trials are necessary to define the role of n-3 fats further in psychiatry.

Lovaza® is a prescription form of n-3 fats in the United States indicated for the treatment of hypertriglyceridemia. Please see the PDR entry for full details. The suggested dose of this medication for its indication is 4g per day of EPA and DHA in a ratio of 1:0.81. In hepatic impairment, alanine aminotransferase and aspartate aminotransferase should be monitored. Low-density lipoprotein cholesterol should also be monitored because it may increase with rapid decreases in triglycerides. This medication may be contraindicated when fish allergies are present. Adverse events include GI upset, fishy aftertaste, rash, and pruritus.

This medication may increase bleeding time but not beyond normal limits. Bleeding time should be monitored if the patient is receiving concurrent anticoagulant medication. This medication is pregnancy category C: Animal-reproduction studies show an adverse effect on fetuses, and there have been no adequate and well-controlled studies in humans, but potential benefits may warrant use in pregnant women despite potential risks. In pregnant rats, five times the human dose is not hazardous. Use caution when breastfeeding. This medication has not been studied in the pediatric population. Safety and efficacy in subjects older than 60 years is not different from those in subjects younger than 60 years. Women have greater uptake of n-3 fats into phospholipids than do men. There is no carcinogenicity in rats at up to five times the human dose for 89 to 110 weeks. There are no adverse effects on rat fertility at up to five times the human dose. On the basis of the EPA:DHA ratio, Lovaza® is a suitable (but not ideal) source of n-3 fats for the treatment of ADHD. It would be preferable to use a product with a higher EPA:DHA ratio.

In addition to supplementing with EPA, preliminary evidence suggests that the addition of GLA may improve symptoms of inattention associated with ADHD.[242] Although GLA itself and the common sources of GLA, borage and evening primrose oil, do not have GRAS status granted by the FDA, other sources of GLA, including spirulina[243] and oils from *Buglossoides arvensis* seeds,[244] do have this designation. Concerns have been raised over the possibility of increased seizure risk in those taking evening primrose oil[245]; however, further investigation into these reports and more recent research suggest that these claims are spurious and that GLA may act as an anticonvulsant.[246] Therefore, a history of seizures may no longer be a contraindication to taking evening primrose oil. Borage and possibly other sources of GLA may not be safe in pregnancy, as there may be risk of fetal harm and induction of early labor.[247] Possible adverse effects of evening primrose oil include headache, abdominal pain, nausea, and loose stools.[248] Clients who have or are at risk of prostate cancer are advised to avoid the use of GLA and n-6 fats in general because this may increase risk or exacerbate the condition.[249] GLA has the potential to interact with several medications, including anticoagulants (potentiation), antibiotics (ceftazidime; may increase effectiveness), immunosuppressants (cyclosporine; may increase effectiveness and protect against associated kidney damage), and several anticancer medications (potentiation).[250] Given the current evidence, it may make the most sense to supplement with borage oil containing 240 to 300mg of GLA per softgel until GLA from other sources is more readily available.

Recommended Brands of High-Potency Omega-3 Softgels:
Thorne Super EPA Pro contains EPA 650mg and DHA 100mg per softgel.

Vitamin Shoppe Omega-3 Fish Oil 735 EPA contains EPA 735mg and DHA 165mg per softgel.

NutriGold triple strength fish oil contains EPA 725mg and DHA 250mg per softgel.

Recommended Brands of High-Potency Omega-3 Liquid:
Nordic Naturals Ultimate Omega XTRA contains EPA 2000mg and DHA 1000mg per *teaspoon* (when very high doses of 5-10g every day are attempted, this may be the best choice).

Barlean's Ultra High Potency Omega Swirl contains EPA 540mg and DHA 540mg per *1 tablespoon*, which is *3 teaspoons* (apparently does not taste fishy at all).

Vegan sourced DHA and EPA (produced from yeast) by Pure Encapsulations.

Magnesium and Vitamin B6

Magnesium and vitamin B6 at a glance:

May address: Inattention, hyperactivity, aggression; anecdotal for sleep

Dose: 6-9mg/kg divided twice a day, with larger dose at bedtime

Time to onset of action: 30-60 minutes for sedative effects; 2-4 months for ADHD symptoms

AEs: Sedation and loose stools, see full PDR entry

GRAS: Yes

Possible MOA: Neurotransmitter and essential fatty acid synthesis, GABAergic, serotonergic

Magnesium is a trace element essential to all cells of all known living organisms. Vitamin B6 (pyridoxine) is a water-soluble nutrient necessary for numerous metabolic processes, including the production of the key neurotransmitters: serotonin, epinephrine, norepinephrine, and GABA.[251]

Evidence for the Efficacy of Magnesium and Vitamin B6 in Treating ADHD

Correlations exist between ADHD symptoms, especially hyperactivity and decreased Mg levels in red blood cells (RBCs).[252] Of 116 children with ADHD, 95% were magnesium deficient in serum (33.6%), RBCs (58.6%), and/or hair (77.6%).[253] Three open-label studies in a total of 142 children with ADHD given magnesium (6mg/kg/d or 200mg/d) alone and with vitamin B6 (0.6mg/kg/d) for one to six months found significant improvements in hyperactivity, aggression, and attention.[254] After at least two months of treatment, hyperactivity, school attention, and aggression all improved ($p < 0.0001$).[255]

When magnesium and B6 were discontinued, symptoms reappeared within a few weeks. Hyperactivity improved after two months of treatment ($p<0.05$), with greater efficacy after four months ($p<0.001$).[256] Aggression and inattention improved after four months of treatment ($p<0.01$) but not at earlier assessments.[257] Wender's behavior scale ($p<0.01$), Quotient of Development to Freedom from Distractibility ($p<0.001$), and CPRS and CTRS ($p<0.001$) scores all improved significantly.[258]

Evidence for the efficacy of B6 in treating ADHD independently of magnesium is indirect and anecdotal. A recent study posited that quantities and ratios of B6-dependent metabolic reactions could serve as biomarkers for the disorder.[259] Urine samples of treated (methylphenidate) and untreated children with ADHD compared with those of controls revealed imbalances in metabolites of the B6-dependent reactions involved in the metabolism of the amino acid tryptophan, which could be reflective of inborn errors of B6 metabolism. The authors concluded that the activity of B6-dependent enzymes of tryptophan degradation are dramatically impaired in ADHD. These impairments are partially, but not fully, ameliorated by treatment with methylphenidate. They further stated that long-term (years) B6 treatment is safe and effective for treating ADHD, with behavior normalizing within several weeks and symptoms returning within one or two months of stopping treatment.[260] However, no specific evidence or statistics are given to support these claims.

Metadoxine is an ion-pair salt of vitamin B6[261,262] and is a precursor to the metabolically active form, pyridoxal 5'-phosphate (P5P). It has been used for more than 30 years for acute alcohol intoxication and alcohol withdrawal syndrome.[263] Recent controlled trials have shown the extended release version may be effective in the treatment of adults with ADHD both short term[264] and over a six-week period.[265,266] Metadoxine as a form of B6 may play a role in the metabolism of neurotransmitters central to the presence and amelioration of ADHD symptoms. Animal studies indicate that it increases levels of dopa-mine,[267] GABA, and acetylcholine[268] in certain brain regions. Additional well-designed studies are necessary to elucidate the role of various forms of B6 in the treatment of ADHD.

How to Prescribe Magnesium and B6 for ADHD

Use Mg citrate, Mg glycinate, Mg taurate, or Mg threonate weight based at 6mg per kilogram of body weight per day, along with vitamin B6 (preferably in the activated form, P5P) weight based at 0.6mg per kilogram of body weight per day. Be aware that two to four months may be required for maximum effect. Higher doses of magnesium may be necessary for clin-ical response. Like benzodiazepines, magnesium is a GABA A receptor agonist.[269] It also may increase levels of serotonin[270] and may have mood-stabilizing properties.[271] Improvement in core symptoms, such as hyperactivity, aggression, and inattention, have been observed when magnesium is supple-mented with and without vitamin B6.[272]

Magnesium may cause daytime sedation. If this occurs, part of the dose or the entire dose may be given at bedtime. Magne-sium may also be effective for insomnia and sleep problems associated with ADHD. Vitamin B6 has many roles in human metabolism, including the conversion of plant-based n-3 fats to EPA and DHA, as well as amino acid metabolism and the production of serotonin, GABA, dopamine, and norepineph-rine. Mg citrate liquid is indicated as a laxative for constipation and bowel preparation prior to colonoscopy. Please see entire product insert for prescribing guidelines.

The amount of the dose of Mg citrate liquid absorbed in adults may be as high as 2800mg; in children six to 12 years old, 1163mg; and in children two to six years old, 140mg. Adverse events may include palpitations, dizziness, fainting, GI cramping, diarrhea, nausea, vomiting, bloating, flatulence, sweating, and weak-ness. Pregnancy category and safety during lactation are unde-termined. Avoid use in patients with renal dysfunction because it may lead to hypermagnesemia. Note that doses of Mg citrate liquid are significantly higher than amounts suggested for treatment of ADHD. Pyridoxine hydrochloride is prescribed intramuscularly or intravenously for dietary deficiency, medication-induced deficiency (due to isoniazid or birth control pill use), and inborn errors of metabolism (B6-dependent convulsions and B6-responsive anemia). Please see PDR entry for full prescribing considerations. Recommended daily allowance in adults is 2.2mg, and 2.5mg during pregnancy and lactation. It may antagonize the effects of L-dopa, but not if L-dopa is taken with carbidopa. Requirements are increased when patients are taking birth control pills. B6 is pregnancy category A and may be useful for nausea and vomiting.

Adverse events may include paresthesia, somnolence, and low serum folate levels. Symptoms of dependence have been reported in adults taking megadoses of 200mg per day. Doses of 25mg per day in adult humans are well tolerated. Very high doses may exceed the liver's ability to convert B6 to its active form, P5P, leading to high levels of B6, which may be directly neurotoxic or compete with P5P for binding sites, thereby causing a relative deficiency.[273] Neurotoxicity is associated with doses of at least 500mg per day for two years.[274] P5P has not been associated with toxicity.[275]

Dietary Modifications to Increase Intake of Magnesium and Vitamin B6

Levels of RBC Mg have been found to be significantly decreased in ADHD. Both magnesium and B6 may improve core symptoms when they are increased via diet or supplementation. Low levels of dietary magnesium and B6 may be caused by how the food we choose is processed, refined, packaged, and stored. For example, unrefined wheat is a good source of magnesium, but refined wheat has only 16% of the magnesium remaining.[276] Similarly, storage, processing, freezing, and canning may destroy 30% to 70% of the vitamin B6 in foods. Increasing dietary intake of spices, nuts, cereals, cocoa, tea, and green leafy vegetables is a good way to counter low levels of magnesium. Meat, whole grains, vegetables, nuts, and bananas are all good sources of B6.

Suggested Use:
Anecdotally, Mg in various forms, including Mg citrate, Mg glycinate, Mg taurate, Mg threonate, and Mg orotate, with weight-based dosing at 6 to 9mg per kilogram of body weight at bedtime, may be effective for sleep problems associated with ADHD.

Zinc
Zinc at a glance:

May address: Optimize therapeutic effects of stimulants, decrease affective blunting associated with stimulants

Dose: Age based (see full details in text), twice daily dosing is preferable

Time to onset of action: Possibly 3-5 weeks

AEs: See PDR

GRAS: Yes

Prescription forms: Yes

Possible MOA: Neurotransmitter and essential fatty acid synthesis

Zinc is an essential trace element necessary for plants, animals, and microorganisms.

Evidence for the Efficacy of Zinc in Treating ADHD
In a study in 43 six- to 12-year-old Canadian children with ADHD, 66% were found to have a serum zinc deficiency. Interestingly, no correlation was found between dietary zinc intake and serum zinc status.[277] These findings suggest that there may be greater zinc turnover or elimination in subjects with

ADHD. Both zinc and methylphenidate are dopamine transporter inhibitors. Response rates to stimulant medications are decreased if zinc serum levels are low.[278] A randomized controlled study in 52 US children with ADHD receiving zinc glycinate 15mg every morning or twice per day for eight weeks found that it was ineffective for improving symptoms.[279]

However, zinc along with d-amphetamine for five weeks resulted in a 37% decrease in the dose of the stimulant medication required and reduced affective blunting from the stimulant medication from 21% in the placebo group to 11% in the zinc group. Zinc given in the morning may be excreted by afternoon but while in the system tends to improve symptoms of ADHD and may act similarly to an immediate-release stimulant.

How to Prescribe Zinc for ADHD:
Ideally, zinc should be prescribed only if there is evidence of deficiency on laboratory test results. Zinc glycinate or gluconate produces less GI upset than zinc sulfate and may be more absorbable. For children four to eight years old, use 5 to 12mg per day, ideally divided twice a day (morning and early afternoon); for children nine to 13 years old, use 8 to 23mg per day; for those 14 to 18 years old, use 11 to 34mg per day; and for those 19 years or older, use 11 to 40mg per day. Zinc is required for the metabolism of dopamine, melatonin, and omega fats.[280] Deficiency has been observed in ADHD,[283] and this may be independent of levels of dietary intake. Zinc may optimize the therapeutic effects of stimulant medications, allowing for a lower dose of these medications and decreasing the affective blunting associated with stimulants.[282] Be aware that zinc is generally included in most multivitamins, and this additional amount should be taken into account. Zinc sulfate 5mg/ml is indicated for zinc deficiency in total parenteral nutrition. See full PDR entry. Zinc administration in the absence of copper may decrease serum copper levels, so periodic monitoring is suggested.

Dietary Modifications to Increase Intake of Zinc:
Zinc deficiency has been significantly associated with ADHD symptoms. Correcting this deficiency may improve ADHD symptoms and allow for lower doses of stimulant medications, as well as fewer side effects. It is found in high amounts in oysters, lobster, red meat, and liver. Going out to an oyster bar for breakfast or serving liver in the morning probably would not go over well. Therefore, if levels are found to be low, using supplements may be a more reasonable approach.

Iron
Iron at a glance:

May address: Inattention, hyperactivity, conduct problems, anxiety if ferritin levels are low; may allow for lower dose of stimulant medication

Dose: Weight based and time limited if ferritin levels are low (see full details in text)

AEs: Constipation with some formulations, see PDR

GRAS: Yes

Prescription forms: Yes

Possible MOA: Neurotransmitter synthesis, dopamine transporter expression

Iron is an essential trace element found in nearly all living organisms.

Evidence for the Efficacy of Iron in the Treatment of ADHD
Ferritin is an intracellular protein that stores and releases iron in a controlled way. The amount of ferritin in the serum reflects the amount of stored iron in the body. Iron is an essential trace mineral required for numerous metabolic processes, many of which directly affect neurologic function. It is necessary for the synthesis of serotonin, dopamine, and norepinephrine, as well

as the activity of the enzyme monoamine oxidase (MAO). Iron deficiency is associated with decreased dopamine transporter expression.[283] A number of studies have examined the relationship between iron status and ADHD presence and severity.

Some evidence has failed to show an association,[284,285,286] whereas other findings suggest that low serum ferritin levels correlate significantly with ADHD.[287,288,289,290] A randomized controlled study in 52 US children with ADHD found that low serum ferritin levels were correlated with inattention, hyperactivity and impulsivity, total ADHD scores, and a higher dose of stimulant medication needed for a therapeutic response.[291] A study in 118 seven- to 14-year-olds with ADHD found that decreased ferritin was associated with increased CPRS total, conduct problems, and increased anxiety and hyperactivity scores.[292] Out of a sample of 60 children with ADHD, 63.3% of those with the inattentive subtype had low levels of serum ferritin, which was significantly greater than in other subtypes. Moreover, five out of nine of those with the inattentive subtype with low ferritin levels had a complete response, and three out of nine had a partial response when treated with supplemental iron for three months, whereas seven out of eight with other subtypes of ADHD (not inattentive) did not respond to supplemental iron.[293] One study also suggested an association between parent-reported sleep difficulties in children with ADHD and low ferritin levels.[294] Although additional research is needed to explore this relationship, ferritin levels should be included in the overall evaluation of children with ADHD,[295] and when levels are deficient, they should be corrected with supplemental iron.

How to Prescribe Iron for ADHD
Iron should be supplemented only in patients with low serum ferritin levels. Low levels have been correlated with inattention, hyperactivity, impulsivity, conduct problems, anxiety, and total ADHD scores, as well as higher doses of stimulant medication needed for therapeutic response.[296,297] Use ferrous

sulfate, gluconate, or fumarate weight based in children 3 to 6mg per kilogram of body weight per day and 60mg per day in adolescents. Treat for one month and then recheck levels. Continue treatment for two to three months after laboratory test result levels are corrected. Then recheck every six months. See full prescribing details. GI adverse events are usually dose related and include nausea, constipation, anorexia, vomiting, and dark stools. Minimize adverse effects by starting with a low dose and titrating upward. A suggested iron supplement is Floradix, a plant-based liquid iron supplement that has a reputation for being nonconstipating, unlike other iron supplements.

Dietary Modifications to Increase Intake of Iron

Iron deficiency, as indicated by low levels of ferritin, has been correlated with core symptoms of ADHD and the need for higher doses of stimulant medication. Iron-rich foods include red meat, egg yolks, leafy greens, prunes and raisins, oysters, clams, scallops, beans, liver, and artichokes. Incorporating such foods into our diets can obviate the need for supplementation.

Vitamin D3

Vitamin D3 at a glance:

May address: No direct evidence for efficacy in ADHD

Dose: Only supplemented if 25-hydroxyvitamin D levels are low (see full details in text)

AEs: See PDR

Vitamin D refers to a group of fat-soluble substances that are necessary for a number of metabolic processes, including intestinal absorption of calcium and phosphate. Cholecalciferol (D3) and ergocalciferol (D2) are the most important D vitamins in humans. Although it is commonly referred to as a vitamin, technically it is not, as the term *vitamin* refers to essential substances that cannot be synthesized in sufficient quantities by an organism. D vitamins can be synthesized from cholesterol upon exposure to adequate sunlight.

Evidence for the Efficacy of Vitamin D3 in the Treatment of ADHD

Three recent studies examining vitamin D levels in children with ADHD from Quata and Turkey have found significant correlations between the diagnosis and low serum levels.[298,299,300] However, results from these studies may not be applicable to US populations. Although there are no studies directly examining the effects of vitamin D deficiency or supplementation on symptoms of ADHD, evidence suggests that there are links between vitamin D and cognitive and behavioral functioning. It is involved in both brain development and function and appears to have significant neuroprotective and anti-inflammatory effects.[301] However, few studies directly examine cognitive and behavioral functional end points, and the results are suggestive as opposed to definitive.[302] Vitamin D is recommended for protection against rickets, bone fracture risk, and possibly some forms of cancer.[303]

How to Prescribe Vitamin D for ADHD

Vitamin D in the form of vitamin D3 should be supplemented in patients who have low levels as indicated by laboratory test results. Serum levels should be greater than 20ng/ml, but 32ng/ml may be the true limit for sufficiency. When levels are very low, supplemental doses of up to 5000 units per day may be required. It is suggested that at supplemental doses greater than 400 units per day (the minimum daily requirement), 30 to 75mg of elemental calcium be prescribed daily (this translates to approximately 150-350mg of calcium citrate). One to two weeks after starting vitamin D therapy, this dose of calcium may be decreased by 50%. Vitamin D levels should then be rechecked after three months and then annually.[304] Symptoms of vitamin D toxicity include anorexia, polyuria, and heart arrhythmias. This is unlikely to occur at doses below 10000 units per day but over time may lead to blood levels greater than 125 to 150ng/

ml, which should be avoided. Blood levels greater than 200ng/ml are considered toxic.[305] Refer to the US National Library of Medicine MedlinePlus website at https://ods.od.nih.gov/fact-sheets/VitaminD-Consumer/#h10 for important information about medication interactions.

Dietary Modifications to Increase Intake of Vitamin D
Foods naturally rich in vitamin D include certain species of fish like salmon, mackerel, and herring; eggs; liver; and some mushrooms like button and shiitake. Dairy products and milk substitutes are often enriched with vitamin D.

Probiotics
Probiotics at a glance:

May address: Indirect evidence of efficacy in addressing increased oxidative stress associated with ADHD, allergic rhinitis associated with ADHD, and food allergies associated with ADHD

Dose: At least 5-10 billion colony-forming units (CFUs) of broad-spectrum probiotics daily

AEs: See full details in text

GRAS: Yes, some strains (and many more by European standards)

Prescription forms: Yes

Medical food: Yes

Possible MOA: IIO axis

The term *probiotics* refers to microorganisms or bacteria that may be found in the human GI tract, in cultured or fermented foods, and in the environment that confer health benefits to the host when consumed or when present in the body. Hundreds of different species of bacteria inhabit the human GI tract.

Collectively, there are 10 times as many of these cells than our own cells in our bodies, and they possess at least 100 times as many genes as our own DNA.[306] This mass of cells constitutes a virtual inner organ[307] whose functions across evolutionary time and within the life spans of individuals is only beginning to be understood.

Currently, in industrialized countries, there is a predominance of allergic, autoimmune, and chronic inflammatory disorders as opposed to infectious diseases.[308] Allergic disorders affect 15% to 20% of Western populations and have been increasing over the past few decades.[309] It has been hypothesized that environmental factors like improved sanitation, decreased family size, and increased use of antimicrobials and consumption of sterile foods[310] have disrupted the previously inevitable interaction between microorganisms and our developing immune systems, leading to excessive and inappropriate immune responses to antigens in the environment and within the body.

This loss of contact, in turn, may lead to the observed increased rates in allergic, autoimmune, and inflammatory conditions.[311] The human genome may not encode for all of the proteins required for immune system development. Therefore, we have depended on interactions with the collective genomes of the environmental microbiota to shape immune functions. Contact with probiotics throughout our life span can cause immune cells to differentiate along immunoregulatory lines leading to the production of anti-inflammatory cytokines that help induce and maintain an adaptive level of immune suppression.[312] Maturation of immune responses from type 2 helper T cells (Th2) in infancy to increasing type 1 helper T cells (Th1) tends to decrease the development of childhood allergic disorders.[313] Loss of exposure to these benign microorganisms may sensitize certain individuals in industrialized societies to mount inappropriately aggressive inflammatory responses to nonthreatening internal and external factors, leading to autoimmune and inflammatory disorders.[314]

Probiotics are a heterogeneous group of bacteria species with specific characteristics. Potential therapeutic mechanisms of action include aiding in the digestion of food; nutrient absorption; protection against colonization by pathogens; immuno-regulation[315]; improved intestinal barrier function; and making antimicrobial compounds,[316] antioxidants,[317] and enzymes.[318] The efficacy of probiotic therapy depends on numerous factors, including the type of microorganism used, the dose (expressed as the number of CFUs), the length of treatment, and the diet and health status of the host.[319] Inconsistency of findings among studies on probiotics is likely related to differences in selected populations, strains used,[320] and dosing regimens.

Notwithstanding, accumulating evidence suggests that probi-otics possess powerful antioxidant and anti-inflammatory prop-erties,[321] are essential in the development and maintenance of a properly functioning immune system,[322] and may have ther-apeutic effects in a number of medical[323] and psychiatric disor-ders, including autistic spectrum disorders,[324] depression,[325] anxiety,[326] and stress-related disorders,[327] possibly secondary to modulation of gamma-aminobutyric acid (GABA),[328] sero-tonin,[329] cannabinoid,[330] and cortisol[331] and corticosterone[332] systems.

Evidence for the Efficacy of Probiotics in Treating ADHD

Despite the growing body of research on the roles of various probiotics in both healthy and diseased states, currently there are no available studies in the peer-reviewed literature that directly investigate their role in the treatment of ADHD. However, there are several lines of indirect evidence showing by extrapo-lation that certain probiotics may be related to the development and treatment of ADHD. This evidence, when taken together with the favorable risk-to-benefit ratio of probiotics, makes them a recommended essential nutrient for the treatment of ADHD within certain subpopulations and arguably for all clients with the disorder. There is anecdotal evidence that children with ADHD may have a deficit of probiotic bacteria.

Michael R. Lyon, MD, reported in his 2002 book, *Is Your Child's Brain Starving?*,[333] that research he performed in 75 children with ADHD indicated most of the children had little or no friendly gut bacteria, all had high levels of pathogenic bacteria, and about one-third had potentially pathogenic yeast. Specifics of the study, including population characteristics, design, statistical analysis, and other details, were not provided. Additional well-controlled published studies are necessary to corroborate these findings. ADHD is associated with increased oxidative stress,[334] and preliminary evidence suggests that decreasing this oxidative stress, as evidenced by improvements in the biomarkers 8-oxoguanine (8-oxoG) and total antioxidant status (TAS), is positively correlated with improvement in core symptoms of ADHD.[335]

Evidence is accumulating that probiotic supplementation exerts antioxidant effects and improves several biomarkers of oxidative stress, including those that correlate with ADHD symptom improvement.[336] In a randomized single-blind trial, a probiotic-enriched yogurt with *Lactobacillus bulgaricus*, *Streptococcus thermophilus*, *Lactobacillus acidophilus*, and *Bifidobacterium lactis* decreased 8-oxoG ($p<0.04$) during pregnancy, a condition associated with increased oxidative stress.[337] In a randomized controlled trial, probiotic yogurt with *L acidophilus* and *B lactis* increased TAS ($p<0.05$) in subjects with diabetes mellitus type 2.[338]

Malondialdehyde (MDA), another indicator of oxidative stress, is increased in ADHD.[339] In animal models of liver injury[340] and acute pancreatitis,[341] *Lactobacillus paracasei* and a combination of *L acidophilus*, *Lactobacillus casei*, *Lactobacillus salivarius*, *Lactococcus lactis*, *Bifidobacterium bifidum*, and *B lactis*, respectively, significantly lowered MDA. Additionally, in a placebo-controlled trial in athletes, supplementation with *Lactobacillus rhamnosus* and *L paracasei* significantly increased plasma antioxidant levels.[342] Therefore, in some conditions associated with increased oxidative stress, supplementation with certain probiotic strains appears to improve several biomarkers of oxidative stress. It is reasonable to hypothesize that supplementation of these probiotics in clients with ADHD could improve parameters of oxidative stress and, by extension, symptoms of the disorder. Studies designed to investigate this hypothesis are needed to determine whether this is the case. As previously discussed, allergic hypersensitivities, including the presence of allergic rhinitis and food allergies, have been correlated with ADHD. Treating these conditions decreases the predisposition for ADHD symptoms and reduces the need for other interventions.

A number of well-designed studies indicate that several strains of probiotics, including *L acidophilus*,[343] *L bulgaricus*,[344] *L casei*,[345] *Lactobacillus gasseri*,[346] *L paracasei*,[347] *Lactobacillus plantarum*,[348] *L salivarius*,[349] *S thermophilus*,[350] *Bifidobacterium*,[351] and *Bifidobacterium longum*,[352] significantly improve symptoms of allergic rhinitis. A meta-analysis of randomized controlled trials of probiotics for allergic rhinitis[353] concluded that probiotic use resulted in decreased symptom severity, decreased use of medications for the condition, and increased quality of life. These findings were strain specific. Although the literature examining the effects of probiotics on food allergies is less extensive, has focused on animals, and has yielded inconsistent results,[354] several strains, including *L acidophilus*,[355] *Bifidobacterium*,[356] and *B lactis*,[357] have shown positive effects in this regard.

VSL#3 is a high-potency probiotic medical food indicated for the management of ulcerative colitis, irritable bowel syndrome, and ileal pouch.[358] It contains *Bifidobacterium breve*, *B longum*, *Bifidobacterium infantis*, *L acidophilus*, *L plantarum*, *L paracasei*, *L bulgaricus*, and *S thermophilus*. Each packet contains 450 billion CFUs, and each capsule contains 112.5 billion. There is also a prescription (from VSL#3-DS) that contains 900 billion CFUs. This product contains many (but not all) of the strains that would address oxidative stress, allergic rhinitis, and food allergies.

How to Prescribe Probiotics for ADHD

Start with a broad-spectrum probiotic supplement that contains a variety of microorganisms dosed to provide at least 5 billion CFUs in children and 10 billion CFUs in adults given with or shortly after meals for a minimum of two to three weeks. Higher doses may be used for improved clinical response.

Strains that address the increased oxidative stress associated with ADHD include *B lactis, B bifidum, L acidophilus, L bulgaricus, L casei, L lactis, L paracasei, L rhamnosus, L salivarius*, and/or *S thermophilus*. For allergic rhinitis symptoms, use *B longum, L acidophilus, L bulgaricus, L casei, L gasseri, L paracasei, L plantarum, L salivarius*, and/or *S thermophilus*. Food allergy symptoms may be addressed with *L acidophilus* and/or *B lactis*.

It is more convenient to use broad-spectrum products that contain a number of different strains rather than isolated strains. In general, probiotics must be purchased refrigerated and kept cold to ensure the viability of the microorganisms. Most research on probiotics have used between 1 and 20 billion CFUs per day. Doses of more than 5 billion CFUs in children and more than 10 billion CFUs in adults have been associated with better outcomes.[359] These doses for at least five days have also been suggested for successful intestinal colonization to occur.[360] Studies investigating antioxidant and antiallergy effects of probiotics allow several weeks to three months for therapeutic effects to become apparent. It may be advisable to take probiotics with meals or shortly afterward because food dilutes stomach acids, which increases probiotic survival to the intestines.

A large number of probiotics are considered safe and have been approved by the European Food Safety Authority. *B bifidum, B breve, B longum, L acidophilus, Lactobacillus brevis, L casei, L bulgaricus, L gasseri, Lactobacillus helveticus, L paracasei, L plantarum, L rhamnosus*, and *S thermophilus*[361] have all been granted a positive Qualified Presumption of Safety,[362] which is similar to GRAS status in the United States. *S thermophilus, B lactis, L acidophilus,* and *L lactis* have GRAS status in the United States.[363] In a literature review of 622 studies on probiotics, 235 made nonspecific safety statements like "well-tolerated," and 387 reported the presence or absence of one or more specific adverse events. Adverse events were primarily gastrointestinal in nature and included nausea, diarrhea, and constipation.[364]

Probiotics have the potential to cause invasive infections in hosts who have compromised mucosal epithelia. This has mostly been observed in immunocompromised adults. Therefore, either avoid use in these populations or be aware of a risk of sepsis.[365] Case studies have indicated that fungemia, bacteremia, and sepsis may be associated with probiotic supplementation, but parallel randomized controlled trials showed no statistically significant increased risk of serious adverse events. The majority of cases of serious adverse events were in critically ill patients or subjects with multiple morbidities when they contracted serious infections potentially caused by probiotics. A subgroup analysis of all randomized controlled trials enrolling critically ill patients showed no statistically significant risk of adverse events. Additionally, a stratified study indicated no increased risk of adverse events in children, adults, or elderly subjects.[366]

Recommended Probiotic Products:

1. ProThera's Ther-Biotic Complete capsules (25+ billion CFUs per capsule) or powder (25+ billion CFUs per one-sixteenth of a teaspoon): This broad-spectrum product contains *B bifidum, B breve, B lactis, B longum, L acidophilus, L breve, L bulgaricus, L casei, L paracasei, L plantarum, L rhamnosus,* and *S thermophilus.*

2. Ultra Jarro-Dophilus: This broad-spectrum product contains 40 billion CFUs per capsule of *B breve, B lactis, B longum, L acidophilus, L casei, L lactis, L paracasei, L plantarum, L rhamnosus,* and *L salivarius.* It tends to be more widely available than ProThera products.

Multinutrient Approach

A multinutrient approach refers to the combined use of nutrients that individually may have direct efficacy in treating ADHD or may be indirectly helpful for ADHD symptoms by addressing possible deficiencies in metabolic pathways.

Evidence for the Efficacy of a Multinutrient Approach in Treating ADHD

Experiments designed to determine whether a particular medication or nutrient is likely to be effective in treating ADHD, or any other disorder for that matter, endeavor to isolate it as a single intervention. In this way, if a therapeutic effect is found, it can be more confidently associated with the medication or nutrient. However, it has been suggested that researching single nutrients may be too narrow. Vitamins, minerals, and other nutrients affect the absorption and effectiveness of each other.[367] They do not work independently. Rather, they interdependently act to help form the intricate web that makes up our metabolism. ADHD is a complex disorder with heterogeneous symptoms and etiologies. Therefore, it is not surprising that multi-ingredient supplementation may be beneficial.[368] As opposed to the more mixed results from studies on single nutrients, data on multinutrient approaches tend to be more consistently positive.[369]

In a study in 20 seven- to 12-year-olds with ADHD, 10 were prescribed methylphenidate by a family physician (5-15mg two or three times a day), and 10 were given a daily multivitamin/mineral/nutrient supplement.[370] The ingredient list of the supplement was quite extensive and included probiotics, amino acids, antioxidants, L-carnitine (30mg), magnesium glycinate (220-480mg), zinc (9-15mg), EPA (180mg), DHA (120mg), and vitamin B6 in the form of P5P. Both groups showed significant gains in scores on a standardized test, with high reliability and validity in diagnosing and assessing ADHD treatment efficacy and medication titration. No significant differences were found between the two groups.

In an observational longitudinal study, 810 four- to 15-year-olds were given daily doses of EPA (400mg), DHA (40mg), GLA (60mg), magnesium (80mg), and zinc (5mg) for 12 weeks at the discretion of their pediatrician.[371] Reasons for being given the supplement combination were lack of concentration (92.1%), inattention (84.1%), aggression (0.7%), hyperactivity or agitation (5.1%), sleep problems (0.4%), and other (2.6%). Thirty-eight percent were found to have clinically relevant attention deficit. When taking all subjects into account, there was a 33.6% improvement in attention scores; 39.5% had clinically relevant hyperactivity or impulsivity, and 63.1% improved to below threshold scores. When all subjects were taken into account, there was a 28.2% improvement in hyperactivity and impulsivity scores. The Strengths and Difficulties Questionnaire emotional problems subscale decreased 28.1%. Over the 12-week treatment period, the percentage of children with problems falling asleep, not sleeping through the night, and reporting poor sleep quality decreased significantly in each area by more than 40%.

In an open-label trial with natural extension, 14 adults with ADHD and severe mood dysregulation receiving no medications for at least four weeks were given a broad-spectrum multivitamin for eight weeks.[372] Ingredients included vitamin D3 (384 IU), B6 (9.6mg), iron (3.7mg), magnesium (160mg), zinc (12.8mg), and three antioxidants. Seven of the 14 adults were found to have major depressive disorder, three had bipolar II, six had social phobia, three had generalized anxiety disorder, and three had alcohol and/or substance abuse problems. There were significant improvements in ADHD symptoms (inattention, hyperactivity, and impulsivity) according to self-reports and observer reports. Effect sizes were large and clinically meaningful. Using a 30% reduction in ADHD symptoms as clinically significant, 28.7% were significantly improved for inattention, and 71.4% were significantly improved for hyperactivity and impulsivity.

Changes in ADHD symptoms were equivalent to or larger than those reported for methylphenidate or atomoxetine treatments in adult samples. In addition to improvements in ADHD symptoms, there were significant improvements on the Montgomery-Asberg Depression Rating Scale or MADRS (a measure of depressive symptoms), quality of life, overall levels of distress and arousal, and ability to regulate anger. During the natural follow-up, all primary outcome measures were lower for those who remained in the supplement group (n=7) than for those who discontinued (n=6).

A DBPC study investigated the effects of vitamin and mineral supplementation in adults with ADHD over an eight-week period.[373] Forty-two medication-free adults were given a broad-spectrum multivitamin and mineral supplement that included all vitamins (except vitamin K) and 16 minerals, while 38 were given a placebo. Doses of specific nutrients of possible therapeutic value in addressing ADHD symptoms were B6 (36mg), magnesium chelate (600mg), zinc (48mg), vitamin D (1440 IU), iron (13.7mg), and ginkgo biloba (36mg). There were no differences in adverse events or clinically significant changes in laboratory test values. In the multivitamin mineral group, 64.3% (versus 36.8% in the placebo group) had at least a 30% decrease from baseline (p<0.014) on one or more subscales of the Conners' Adult ADHD Rating Scales, and 47.6% in the multivitamin mineral group versus 21.1% in the placebo group (p<0.013) were much or very much improved on the Clinical Global Impression-Improvement scale. Participants in the active treatment group reported improvements in both attention and hyperactivity/impulsivity, but only the latter was also noted by observers. Clinicians did not report significant improvements in the ADHD rating scales, but they did see improvement on global functional scales, suggesting a benefit in a variety of areas of psychological functioning. The authors point out that it is difficult for observers to measure attention as opposed to behavioral changes reliably. Furthermore, although self-reported measures of attention improved significantly, scores in the active treatment group remained elevated, calling into question the clinical significance. In the case of hyperactive/impulsive scales, scores in the multivitamin mineral group were decreased down into the nonclinical range.

How to Prescribe Multinutrients for ADHD

Studies suggest that supplementing with a multinutrient approach, which may include essential minerals, vitamins, n-3 fats, amino acids, antioxidants, and/or probiotics, may be effective in the treatment of ADHD symptoms.[374] Although these types of studies do not isolate nutritional variables, they do provide compelling evidence that such nutrients may work synergistically and effectively to treat symptoms and perhaps underlying causes of ADHD.

In order to provide potentially therapeutic nutrients at the right doses, it is preferable to combine several different supplements, which may include a multivitamin, n-3 fats (EPA), magnesium, antioxidants, and probiotics. When choosing a multivitamin, iron-free products with activated B vitamins and absorbable forms of zinc are preferred. Be careful not to exceed the acceptable upper daily intake levels of fat-soluble vitamins (A, E, D, K) and minerals. It may be difficult to obtain a children's vitamin with activated B vitamins and more absorbable forms of minerals like zinc and magnesium, so prescribing an adult multivitamin to children is acceptable, provided the dose is adjusted for age or weight.

Recommended Multivitamin and Mineral Products:

Both of the following contain activated forms of B vitamins and more absorbable forms of minerals:

1. VitaPrime multivitamin by ProThera

2. Multi t/d by Pure Encapsulations

Chapter 12

Prescribing Metabolic Supplements for ADHD

After concurrent administration of essential nutrients for a reasonable period of time (from three weeks to two months), significant symptoms of ADHD may persist. In this case, it is suggested that metabolic nutrients be prescribed in a serial fashion.

Phosphatidylserine, Acetyl-L-Carnitine, and N-Acetylcysteine

At present, these metabolic supplements include phosphatidylserine, acetyl-L-carnitine, and N-acetylcysteine. An adequate trial of each agent individually should occur, while noting efficacy and adverse events. Then, effective or partially effective interventions may be combined for optimum clinical effects.

Phosphatidylserine (PS)

PS at a glance:

May address: Inattention, hyperactivity, impulsivity, oppositionality, mood dysregulation

Dose: 100-400mg in the morning titrated gradually

Time to onset of action: 2-15 weeks

AEs: May increase dopamine and aggravate psychosis, see full details in text

GRAS: Yes

Medical food: Yes

Possible MOA: IIO axis, membrane-lipid therapy, cholinergic, dopaminergic, glutamate modulation

PS, a naturally occurring phospholipid, is one of the structural components of cell membranes. Our bodies can make some PS, but most of what we need comes from dietary sources. It functions as a cofactor for many enzymes and exerts effects on cell excitability and communication.[375] PS has antioxidant,[376] anti-inflammatory,[377] and immunomodulating[378] properties. Its immunoinhibiting functions may help to prevent autoimmune disease.[379]

PS appears to be cholinergic[380] and increases dopaminergic activity by activating tyrosine hydroxylase (the enzyme that catalyzes the rate-limiting step of catecholamine production)[381] and inhibiting MAO-B (the enzyme that deactivates dopamine).[382] Unlike MAO-A, which metabolizes tyramine, MAO-B does not. Therefore, selective MAO-B inhibitors, such as PS, do not pose a risk for hypertensive crises associated with elevated tyramine levels, and no dietary modifications are necessary. In vitro data indicate that PS increases glutamate binding to AMPA receptors, an action that may result from its ability to alter the lipid composition of synaptic membranes.[383] Amplification of glutamatergic action at AMPA receptors has been associated with symptom improvement in adult ADHD patients.[384] Because of its wide-ranging effects, PS may have additional applications in depression,[385] mild cognitive impairment,[386] and adaptation to stress.[387]

Evidence for the Efficacy of PS in the Treatment of ADHD
PS supplementation targets ADHD symptoms via several mechanisms of action. It is a form of membrane-lipid therapy, addresses IIO axis issues, and modulates AMPA receptors, dopamine and acetylcholine. A pilot study in 15 six- to 12-year-olds with ADHD given PS 200mg per day for two months resulted in significant improvements in ADHD scores ($p<0.01$), inattention scores ($p<0.01$), hyperactivity/impulsivity scores ($p<0.05$), and the number of correct answers on a visual perception task ($p<0.001$).[388] In a DBPC study in 200 children with ADHD, 137 were given PS 300mg per day, EPA 86mg per day, and DHA 34mg

per day for 15 weeks followed by an open-label extension for another 15 weeks.[389] This intervention resulted in a decrease in the global restless/impulsive subscale of the CPRS (p<0.05) and the parent impact-emotional subscale of the Child Health Questionnaire (p<0.05).

The subgroups with increased hyperactivity/impulsivity and mood and behavioral dysregulation showed a decrease in the ADHD index and hyperactivity/impulsivity components of the CTRS (p<0.05). During the open-label extension with 150 children continuing PS supplementation, CPRS improved for hyperactivity, inattention, impulsivity, and total score (p<0.05), and CTRS improved for oppositionality and hyperactivity (p<0.05). A total of 140 children continued the PS for 30 weeks without any adverse finding on blood test results, blood pressure, heart rate, height, and weight.[390] It was concluded that PS was safe and well tolerated in children.

A randomized controlled trial published in 2014 provides further evidence of the efficacy of PS in addressing ADHD symptoms.[391] Nineteen treatment-naïve four- to 14-year-old children with ADHD were given PS 200mg per day for two months, and 17 were given placebo. The intervention was well tolerated without adverse effects. Overall ADHD symptoms, inattention, and hyperactivity all improved compared with baseline (p<0.01) and so did short-term auditory memory (p<0.05). No significant improvements were observed in the placebo group. These improvements were deemed clinically significant and were associated with improved functioning and quality of life at school and home. The intervention was well tolerated, and no adverse events were reported.

How to Prescribe PS for ADHD
Start with 100mg every morning or 100mg twice a day (morning and early afternoon), then titrate slowly up to a total daily dose of 400mg, if necessary. Higher doses of up to 700mg every day

may be used in some cases. The literature suggests[392] that 15 weeks is necessary to achieve a clinical response, but in practice, results may be seen in two to three weeks. Preliminary evidence suggests that PS is possibly effective for hyperactivity and impulsivity, as well as mood and behavioral dysregulation symptoms. It may be activating, so use caution when clients are using stimulants, and avoid late in the day dosing (and possibly even afternoon dosing) if activation leads to insomnia.

PS may increase dopamine and aggravate psychotic symptoms,[393] so be aware of any history of psychosis and/or mania in the client or family and avoid use in schizophrenia. PS from fish sources has GRAS status granted by the FDA in 2009.[394] Vayarin is a prescription medical food for the clinical dietary management of certain lipid imbalances associated with ADHD.[395] Each capsule contains Lipirinen 167mg, which is composed of PS 75mg, EPA 21.5mg, and DHA 8.5mg. Vayacog, which contains PS, is a medical food indicated for early memory impairment. It is intended to be administered under medical supervision at doses not to exceed 300mg per day. PS is found in meats and fish, especially mackerel, herring, and eel, as well as eggs, soy, and milk. The estimated daily dietary intake is 75 to 184mg. After an oral dose, it appears in the blood within 30 minutes, and plasma levels peak within one to four hours.[396] It crosses the blood-brain barrier and tends to have an affinity for the hypothalamus.[397]

As plant and animal sourced PS have the same metabolic profile, safety profiles are unlikely to be different. Human studies with more than 1500 subjects on doses ranging from 200 to 800mg per day for up to six months show high tolerability without significant adverse events. Some GI upset was noted in high doses greater than 300 to 400mg per day and sleeplessness at doses greater than 600mg per day when taken before bedtime. GI upset is minimized by taking it with food. There are no reported medication, supplement, food, or herbal interactions. PS administered to rats at up to 200mg per kilogram of body weight per day and rabbits at up to 450mg per kilogram of body weight per day showed no effect on embryonic or fetal development. There is no evidence of genetic or bone marrow toxicity. The dose that is lethal in rats 50% of the time, or LD50, is greater than 5g/kg.[398] PS is available from a number of sources, most commonly being supplied in small softgels that contain 100mg each along with other phospholipids (phosphatidylcholine and phosphatidylethanolamine), which naturally co-occur with PS.

Acetyl-L-Carnitine (ALCAR) and L-Carnitine

ALCAR at a glance:

May address: Inattention, hyperactivity; addresses irritability and headaches associated with stimulant medications

Dose: 500-3000mg in the morning

Time to onset of action: Approximately 6 weeks (possibly less)

AEs: Increased dopamine may exacerbate mania and psychosis, possible neuroendocrine and hormonal effects; see full details in the text and PDR entry

GRAS: Yes

Prescription forms: Yes

Possible MOA: IIO axis, membrane-lipid therapy, cholinergic, dopaminergic, noradrenergic, serotonergic

ALCAR is a naturally occurring derivative of L-carnitine, a substance found in foods and made by the body. ALCAR, having anti-inflammatory and antioxidant properties,[399] is effective at decreasing levels of oxidized DNA nucleotides[400] and lipid peroxidation.[401] The former has been associated with improved inattention in ADHD,[402] and the latter may have a role in maintaining membrane integrity. Indeed, ALCAR affects the molecular dynamics of the membrane bilayer, which may be relevant for the expression of membrane function.[403] It affects a number of ADHD-associated neurotransmitter systems, including cholinergic, dopaminergic, norepinephrine, and serotonin.

ALCAR increases the synthesis[404] and release[405] of acetylcholine and prevents the age-related loss of choline acetyltransferase (the enzyme needed to make acetylcholine), thereby potentially rescuing cholinergic pathways from age-associated degeneration.[406] It causes increased norepinephrine release in the hippocampal formation[407] and increased dopamine release in the striatum (nucleus accumbens),[408] and in response to electrical stimulation in aged animals.[409] However, it does not appear to affect the dopamine release evoked by amphetamine,[410] suggesting that adjunctive use of ALCAR with stimulants would be ineffective.

Serotonergic actions include increased levels of serotonin in the nucleus accumbens[411] and cortex,[412] activation of $5\text{-}HT_{1A}$ receptors,[413] and potentiation of both excitatory and inhibitory serotonergic responses.[414] ALCAR plays an integral role in mitochondrial metabolism and notably exhibits neuroprotective activity in a number of potentially neurotoxic environments.[415] It has putative antiaging[416] and antistress[417] effects. Given ALCAR's wide range of actions, it follows that research indicates possible efficacy in the management of several psychiatric and medical conditions, including ADHD, depression,[418] substance abuse,[419] dementia,[420] diabetes,[421] chronic fatigue syndrome,[422] fibromyalgia,[423] and amyotrophic lateral sclerosis.[424]

Evidence for the Efficacy of ALCAR and L-Carnitine in the Treatment of ADHD

Oral ALCAR supplementation targets ADHD symptoms via several mechanisms of action. It addresses specific types of oxidative stress; is a form of membrane-lipid therapy; and modulates cholinergic, dopaminergic, norepinephrine, and serotonergic neurotransmission. A randomized controlled study in 26 boys with ADHD receiving L-carnitine 100mg per kilogram of body weight per day to a maximum dose of 4000mg per day for eight-week intervals alternated with placebo found that on Child Behavior Checklist (CBCL) scores, 13 of the 26 were responders (>30% decrease in scores) (p<0.02).[425] On the CTRS, 12 of the 26 were responders (>30% decrease in the number of most severe ratings) (p<0.02). Responders showed decreases in CBCL total scores (p<0.0001) and subscores for attention (p<0.0001), delinquency (p<0.01), and aggression (p<0.0001). After treatment with L-carnitine, plasma-free carnitine (p<0.03) and ALCAR (p<0.05) levels were higher in responders than in nonresponders. This may indicate that the body converts dietary L-carnitine to ALCAR, which may have superior antioxidant activity within the CNS.[426] At the conclusion of the study, 20 of 24 boys continued L-carnitine at parental request. Six months later, 19 of 20 were judged by parents and teachers to be exhibiting normal (nonclinical) behavior.

A randomized controlled multicenter study in 112 five- to 12-year-olds with ADHD who were receiving ALCAR 500 to 1500mg per day on the basis of body weight for 16 weeks found improvement on the CTRS-R in the ADHD inattentive subtype only (p<0.02), with no significant improvement in the ADHD combined subtype.[427] A randomized controlled study in 40 seven- to 13-year-olds with ADHD who were receiving methylphenidate (20-30mg per day) plus ALCAR (500-1500mg per day) versus methylphenidate plus placebo for six weeks found no significant differences between groups, with both groups showing decreased scores on both parent and teacher rating scales (p<0.001).[428] However, headache and irritability were significantly higher in the group receiving methylphenidate plus placebo. Short study duration, small sample size, and possible overshadowing stimulant doses were likely at play in this study. Two randomized controlled studies on subjects with fragile X syndrome (a genetic disorder strongly associated with ADHD symptoms) who were receiving ALCAR long term (one year) showed significant improvements in behavior.[429]

How to Prescribe ALCAR for ADHD

Start with 500mg every morning and titrate slowly up to 1500mg every morning or more (possibly up to 3000mg every morning). Evidence suggests that ALCAR may be effective for ADHD symptoms, including inattention and hyperactivity,[430] in various populations. It does not appear to be effective as an adjunctive treatment with stimulant medication, but it may decrease the irritability and headaches associated with these medications.

Adverse events, including GI upset, diarrhea, nausea, and vomiting, should be monitored when starting ALCAR and during dose increases. This supplement tends to be stimulating, and caution is advised when it is used in combination with other stimulating medications or supplements. Evidence from animal and human studies suggests that ALCAR may have neuroendocrine and hormonal effects. In vitro, it increases the energy metabolism of rat sertoli cells[431] and increases the secretion of gonadotropin-releasing hormone.[432]

In rats, ALCAR prevents the decreased testosterone that is associated with chronic stress and increased luteinizing hormone (LH) and prolactin.[433] Women with stress-induced amenorrhea and low levels of LH who took 1g of ALCAR per day for 16 weeks had restored LH levels. The intervention had no effect on LH in women with normal levels at baseline.[434] On the basis of available information, it is unclear what effect, if any, supplemental ALCAR may have on hormonal function in adults and children.

Although the PDR does not suggest caution or monitoring in this regard, it may be prudent to monitor testosterone, LH, and prolactin periodically, especially in pediatric cases. It is also noteworthy that ALCAR inhibits the action of the enzyme alcohol dehydrogenase,[435] which is the first step in the metabolism of ethanol (alcohol). Therefore, patients who use alcohol should be advised that their bodies may metabolize drinks more slowly and tolerance may decrease significantly. Typical Western diets provide 100 to 300mg of carnitine per day, mainly depending upon the amount of beef consumed.[436] ALCAR has GRAS status granted by the FDA.[437] It is formed intracellularly (within cells) during normal metabolism in the brain, liver, and kidneys.[438] ALCAR crosses the blood-brain barrier and has a half-life of 4.2 hours. It is minimally metabolized and excreted in the urine. It is considered safe and without serious adverse events even in long-term administration up to one year. The most common adverse events are agitation, nausea, and vomiting. There is one case report of psychosis in a patient with bipolar disorder, possibly secondary to ALCAR's ability to increase dopamine.[439]

ALCAR is available in 500mg capsules from a number of different suppliers. Carnitor is a prescription form of L-carnitine in the United States indicated for the treatment of primary and secondary carnitine deficiency. Please see the PDR entry for full prescribing details. It is important to note that seizures have been reported in patients with and without previous history of seizure. When a history of seizure is present, Carnitor may increase the frequency and/or severity. Caution is advised in this regard. Nicetile has been a prescription form of ALCAR in Italy since 1984 and is indicated for the treatment of mechanical and inflammatory lesions of the peripheral nerve trunk or root.[440] It may be administered orally, intramuscularly, or intravenously and has no risk of addiction or dependence. It also has no known adverse reactions with other medications. Adverse events may include sporadic mild excitement that subsides rapidly with a decreased dose. It is deemed nonhazardous on the basis of human administration safety studies examining repeated dose toxicity, genotoxicity, carcinogenicity, and reproductive toxicity.

Case Study E

A 10-year-old girl recently received a diagnosis of ADHD inattentive subtype with mild symptoms of hyperactivity. Her parents had suspected she had ADHD for approximately three years, with symptoms building to the point of need for intervention. They were opposed to using any prescription medications and were quite motivated in this regard. Prior to the girl being evaluated, her parents had researched the subject of treating ADHD without medications. For one year, they had increased her protein intake in the morning and improved the nutritional profile of her breakfast. This resulted in some minor improvements in symptoms. For approximately three weeks before her assessment, she had been taking the following:

One multivitamin daily

Phosphatidylserine: 70mg per day

Dimethylaminoethanol: 50mg

GABA: 100mg

Lemon balm: 200mg

Chamomile: 50mg

Omega-3 fats: almost exclusively ALA and DHA

Zinc: 14mg per day

Acetyl-L-carnitine: 250mg per day

N-acetyl-L-tyrosine: 300mg per day

Magnesium citrate: 150mg in the morning intermittently

Whey protein: 34g per day

Pycnogenol: 35mg per day

The following recommendations were made initially:

Add EPA 1500mg per day

Increase magnesium citrate 150 to 400mg at bedtime

Add a probiotic supplement (Ultra Jarro-Dophilus)

Hold multivitamin and zinc until laboratory test results come back

Increase phosphatidylserine 100 to 300mg in the morning—titrating slowly

Continue morning smoothies with whey protein

The client was seen two months later when laboratory tests were completed. Her parents reported significant improvements in core symptoms of inattention and hyperactivity, but the remaining symptoms were still problematic. They had continued to give her 35mg of pycnogenol daily.

Laboratory test results revealed a vitamin D level of 30ng/ml, which is the lower end of the normal range. All other laboratory test results were within normal limits. The following recommendations were then made:

Add vitamin D3 at 2000 units per day for several weeks

Continue 1500mg EPA per day

Switch to better-absorbed form of magnesium (she had been taking magnesium oxide); parents decided to switch to magnesium threonate, starting with 144mg at bedtime and titrating slowly to 288mg

Restart multivitamin

Continue probiotic

Continue PS 300mg in the morning

Continue pycnogenol at 35mg per day

At the follow-up six weeks later, the parents reported their daughter had improved significantly and was no longer fidgety at all. Additionally, her grades had improved substantially. The parents felt that there was room for additional improvements with regard to inattentive symptoms and maintaining focus. We discussed adding methylated (activated) forms of B vitamins, as well as either increasing pycnogenol to 70mg per day OR adding a small dose of ALCAR (250mg). Several weeks later, the following supplement regimen was providing adequate control of ADHD symptoms and was continued for the past nine months with continued efficacy and no adverse effects:

One Flintstone multivitamin in the morning

Ultra Jarro-Dophilus: one capsule in the morning

ALCAR: 500mg in the morning

PS: 300mg in the morning

Pycnogenol: 70mg in the morning

Vitamin D3: 1000 IU in the morning

Magnesium threonate: 144mg in the morning and at bedtime

EPA: 1470mg per day

One methyl B12 lozenge

P5P (activated B6): 100mg

Methylfolate (activated folic acid/B9): 1mg

This case is an excellent example of successfully treating pediatric ADHD with a more typically complex NBP regimen, which included supplements and dietary modifications (increased protein and nutrients, especially at breakfast, as well as elimination or reduction of artificial food additives and pesticides). The family's motivation and organization helped to achieve success.

N-Acetylcysteine (NAC)
NAC at a glance:

May address: Indirect evidence for inattention in systemic lupus erythematosus (SLE) patients only

Dose: 150-2400mg twice daily (morning and early afternoon)

Time to onset of action: Unknown—days to 3 months

AEs: See PDR entry

GRAS: Yes

Prescription forms: Yes

Possible MOA: IIO axis, glutamate modulation

N-acetylcysteine or NAC is the acetylated form of the amino acid L-cysteine that is a precursor to glutathione (an endogenous antioxidant); it crosses the blood-brain barrier and is indicated for the treatment of acetaminophen overdose and as a mucolytic agent.[441]

Evidence for the Efficacy of NAC in the Treatment of ADHD
NAC is a powerful antioxidant[442] and anti-inflammatory agent[443] and has a number of potential medical and psychiatric uses, including the treatment of addiction,[444] bipolar disorder,[445] schizophrenia,[446] Alzheimer's dementia,[447] obsessive-compul-

sive disorder,[448] trichotillomania,[449] compulsive nail biting,[450] and compulsive gambling.[451] One small study has been published examining the effects of supplemental NAC on ADHD symptoms in a population with SLE. However, as is the case with probiotics, much indirect evidence suggests that NAC may be an effective intervention for ADHD. Increased oxidative stress associated with ADHD may be addressed, at least in part, by NAC's antioxidant properties. In vitro, animal, and human studies have indicated that in various situations of elevated oxidative stress, NAC increases total antioxidant status (TAS)[452] and decreases a marker of DNA oxidative stress, 8-oxoguanine.[453] These are actions that have been positively correlated with decreased inattention in children with ADHD.[454]

Additionally, NAC has been shown to decrease levels of malondialdehyde (MDA),[455] another indicator of oxidative stress, which is increased in ADHD.[456] NAC is a potent scavenger of hydrogen peroxide and toxic quinones derived from dopamine metabolism,[457] which is thought to be dysregulated in ADHD. One may hypothesize that supplementation with NAC in clients with ADHD could improve parameters of oxidative stress and, by extension, symptoms of the disorder. Well-designed studies are needed to determine whether this is the case.

Stimulant medications commonly used to treat ADHD may have pro-oxidant effects.[458] They may also contribute to inflammation,[459] immune system dysfunction,[460] and decreased levels of endogenous antioxidants.[461] NAC may protect against stimulant-induced oxidative protein damage,[462] behavioral changes, and neurotoxicity.[463] Further evidence for the efficacy of NAC in treating ADHD comes from its actions as a glutamate modulator. Dysregulation of the glutamate system has been recently implicated in the pathophysiology of ADHD.

High levels of impulsivity have been positively correlated with elevated levels of glutamate in certain brain regions.[464] Research suggests that in treatment-naïve subjects with ADHD, levels of this neurotransmitter are increased in some areas of the brain.[465] Moreover, treatment with either methylphenidate or atomoxetine significantly decreased glutamate in the striatum. This was also true in the prefrontal cortex for atomoxetine only.[466] Through a series of complex actions,[467] NAC appears to decrease glutamate levels in conditions in which the neurotransmitter is elevated, including cocaine addiction.[468] Additional studies are needed to determine whether NAC decreases the elevated glutamate associated with ADHD, thereby reducing impulsivity.

A small randomized controlled trial involving 49 patients with SLE and 46 matched controls was carried out to investigate the effects of supplemental NAC in ADHD symptoms as assessed by means of the ADHD Self-Report Scale (ASRS).[469] Twenty-four patients were randomly assigned to receive either placebo, 2.4g NAC per day, or 4.8g NAC per day for three months. At baseline, ASRS scores for inattention and hyperactivity/impulsivity and combined scores were significantly higher in patients with SLE than in controls. Compared with the placebo group, both groups taking NAC had ASRS combined scores that were decreased ($p<0.037$). Also, inattention scores were decreased in those taking 2.4g per day ($p<0.001$) and 4.8g per day ($p<0.0001$). Data from this study indicate that in a population of patients with SLE who have elevated ADHD scores, NAC dose dependently tended to target inattention symptoms significantly. The dose of 4.8g per day was superior to the dose of 2.4g per day. Additional studies are needed to determine whether NAC is effective in the general population with a diagnosis of ADHD.

How to Prescribe N-Acetylcysteine for ADHD
Start with 150mg twice daily (morning and early afternoon) in children and 300mg twice daily in adults. Then titrate slowly to a maximum dose of 2400mg twice daily. It may take several weeks to months for therapeutic effects to become apparent.

Evidence for NAC's efficacy in treating ADHD is extrapolated from its role as an antioxidant and glutamate modulator and its efficacy in decreasing ADHD symptoms in a population with SLE. NAC may be especially effective in addressing inattentive symptoms associated with ADHD. NAC is naturally occurring in a number of foods, including garlic, onions,[470] asparagus, peppers, and parsley,[471] and it has GRAS status (in the form of L-cysteine)[472] and is indicated for both the treatment of acetaminophen overdose and as a mucolytic agent in respiratory illnesses.

Please consult the PDR for full prescribing considerations. Doses used in most studies on psychiatric disorders range from 600 to 2400mg per day, most commonly divided twice a day. Several weeks to a few months are required to observe significant therapeutic effects. Despite evidence that NAC appears to be safe and well tolerated, with the most common adverse effects of nausea, vomiting, and gastrointestinal upset,[473] there are no long-term studies on safety and efficacy. NAC is rapidly absorbed after oral dosing, with peak plasma levels occurring in one hour. After 12 hours, it is no longer detectable,[474] so it is unlikely to accumulate in the body. It is contraindicated in cases of active peptic ulcer. Infrequent anaphylactic reactions secondary to histamine release with associated rash, pruritus, angioedema, bronchospasm, tachycardia, and blood pressure changes have been reported.[475] NAC is widely available and most commonly is supplied in 600mg capsules.

Chapter 13

Prescribing Herbal Supplements for ADHD

After or interspersed with trials of the metabolic supplements, trials of herbs serially in some populations may be warranted. Please note that herbal supplements are the most complex type of supplements and often have a limited evidence base. Therefore, caution is advised when they are used.

Herbal Supplements to Consider

The following herbs may have efficacy in treating ADHD symptoms: pycnogenol, ginkgo biloba, and a compound herbal preparation consisting of *Paeoniae alba* (white peony), *Withania somnifera* (ashwagandha), *Centella asiatica* (gotu kola), *Spirulina platensis* (spirulina), *Bacopa monnieri* (bacopa), *Melissa officinalis* (lemon balm), *Matricaria chamomilla* (chamomile), and *Passiflora incarnata* (passionflower).

Pycnogenol (Pine Bark Extract)

Pycnogenol at a glance:

May address: Inattention

Dose: 1-2mg per kilogram of body weight in the morning or divided twice daily

Time to onset: May take up to 2 months

AEs: See full details in the text

GRAS: Yes

Possible MOA: Antioxidant, membrane-lipid therapy

Pycnogenol is derived from the pine bark tree, which has been used by Native Americans to make tea and medicine for thousands of years.[476] Its active constituents are also found in peanut skin and grape seed.[477] Its well-established antioxidant[478] (decreases lipid peroxidation[479] and DNA damage),[480] anti-inflammatory,[481] immunomodulating,[482] and membrane-lipid therapy[483] properties make it an effective intervention for a host of medical conditions associated with dysfunction of the IIO axis.

Evidence for the Efficacy of Pycnogenol in the Treatment of ADHD

ADHD symptoms appear to be addressed by pycnogenol's anti-oxidant and membrane-lipid effects. A DBPC study in 24 adults 24 to 53 years old with combined type ADHD who were taking pycnogenol 1mg per pound of body weight per day divided three times per day for three weeks found no significant improvement from the intervention.[484] The authors suggested that pycnogenol may need to be administered for longer than three weeks for clinical effects to become apparent. A subset of participants in this study may have benefited from the intervention, as evidenced by several of them contacting their physicians to continue the intervention after completion of the study, along with clinically significant improvement in some of them during the study. This intervention also may not be as effective in an adult ADHD population as it is in children.

A subsequent study seems to suggest this. A randomized controlled trial in 61 six- to 14-year-olds with ADHD who were receiving pycnogenol 1mg per kilogram of body weight every morning for one month, with 44 in the active group and 17 in the placebo group, found decreases in the Child Attention Problems scale according to teachers, compared with baseline ($p < 0.00014$) and placebo ($p < 0.0067$), which returned to baseline after a one-month washout.[485] CTRS inattention scores also decreased compared with baseline ($p < 0.07$) and placebo ($p < 0.049$). CTRS hyperactivity scores and CPRS scores were not significantly improved. Tests for visual-motor coordination and concentration improved compared with baseline ($p < 0.019$) and placebo ($p < 0.05$). However, high values one month after the washout may indicate learning effects.

Morning-only dosing may have decreased detection of improvements by parents. In additional data presented from this same study,[486] after one month of treatment, oxidized glutathione (a marker of oxidative stress) decreased (p<0.013) and returned toward baseline after the one-month washout. Glutathione (an endogenous antioxidant) increased (p<0.0054) and persisted after the washout (p<0.007). Total antioxidant status (TAS), which is decreased in children with ADHD versus controls, increased slightly, then significantly (p<0.002) after the one-month washout. This finding of delay in improvement of TAS may be related to pycnogenol's stimulation of enzymes that may persist well after it is discontinued. There was a positive correlation between inattention scores and TAS normalizing (p<0.035). Additional data showed that, at the start of the trial, children with ADHD had increased levels of a marker of total DNA damage (8-oxoguanine or 8-oxoG) compared with controls (p<0.001).[487]

After one month of treatment, 8-oxoG decreased compared with baseline (p<0.012) and placebo (p<0.014). After the one-month washout, it increased back toward baseline. A correlation was found between 8-oxoG decreasing and inattention scores improving (p<0.0045). Pycnogenol may protect DNA against free radical damage by direct free radical scavenging, chelation, and/or stimulation of DNA repair.

How to Prescribe Pycnogenol for ADHD

Start with a dose of 1mg per kilogram of body weight per day. This may be maintained for approximately one month. Efficacy may be increased by dividing doses twice a day (every morning and early afternoon) and increasing the dose to 2mg per kilogram of body weight per day or more. The full therapeutic effect may take up to two months or longer. Preliminary evidence suggests that it may be effective for symptoms of inattention in ADHD via its antioxidant properties.[488] It does not appear to have actions on specific neurotransmitters or receptor sites. Improvements in ADHD symptoms significantly correlate with improvements in markers of oxidative stress. Monitor for mild and transitory adverse events, including GI upset, dizziness, nausea, headache, sleepiness, urinary retention or frequency, constipation, and sweating, as well as decreased efficacy of any immunosuppressant medications that may be prescribed.

Pycnogenol has GRAS status granted by the FDA.[489] Extensive research has established safety and tolerability for human consumption[490] for doses ranging from 50 to 450mg per day for up to six months in healthy subjects,[491] as well as in patients with hypertension and diabetes.[492] It is readily absorbed, metabolized, and eliminated in humans,[493] with a maximum concentration of constituents seen at five hours and measurable over 14 hours. A steady state is observed after five days of daily dosing.[494] It may increase the activity of the immune system and, therefore, decrease the effectiveness of any prescribed immunosuppressants.[495] Pycnogenol has no other known interactions with supplements, herbs, or foods.[496]

Recommended Pycnogenol Brand Products:
1. Pure Encapsulations 100mg caps

2. ProThera 50mg caps

3. Life Extension 100mg caps

4. Vitacost 100mg caps

Ginkgo Biloba (GB)
GB at a glance:

May address: Inattention, hyperactivity, anxiety

Dose: 80-200mg per day of standardized extract

Time to onset of action: 4-6 weeks

AEs: Possible endocrine or hormonal effects (see full details in the text)

GRAS: No

Possible MOA: IIO axis, membrane-lipid therapy, cholinergic, dopaminergic, noradrenergic, GABAergic

Ginkgo biloba (GB) has been used medicinally for thousands of years in Chinese medicine.[497] Today, it is one of the most widely used and extensively studied herbal supplements.[498] Several active constituents have been identified, including highly toxic substances.[499] Toxic components are commonly removed from most extracts, but there can be variations in the amount of active principles from batch to batch and manufacturer to manufacturer.[500]

When tested for potency, most GB extracts did not meet the stated amounts of active ingredients. Therefore, it is important to use products that are independently tested and for which active constituents are verified from batch to batch.[501] EGb 761 (aka Tanakan) is the most researched standardized extract of GB that contains specific amounts of active ingredients and undetectable or nearly undetectable levels of toxins,[502] including ginkgolic acid (<5 ppm) and ginkgotoxin.

GB extract has potent antioxidant activities,[503] specifically by influencing genetic expression involved in endogenous antioxidant systems,[504] protecting mitochondria from oxidative stress,[505] and preventing lipid peroxidation[506] and the breakdown of phospholipids,[507] which is detrimental to the functioning of cellular membranes. Animal data indicate that EGb 761 increases the n-3 fat EPA in RBC membranes and decreases saturated fats, thus protecting them from oxidative stress.[508] GB also has anti-inflammatory properties.[509] In a study in 31 poststroke patients, the extract increased total antioxidant status (TAS) and decreased high-sensitivity C-reactive protein,[510] a marker of inflammation. It tends to be immunopotentiating[511] in settings of decreased immune function.[512]

GB extract has repeatedly been shown to protect a number of cell types from damage induced by various toxic substances, radiation, and aging. It specifically protects the integrity of neurons in a variety of potentially damaging settings.[513] One mechanism of this neuroprotection is regulating the release of excitotoxic neurotransmitters,[514] including glutamate[515] and glycine.[516] Moreover, GB extract lowers the levels of the stress hormones corticosterone,[517] corticotropin,[518] and corticotropin-releasing hormone,[519] countering the adverse effects of stress in animal and human[520] studies, including cognitive dysfunction.[521] In rats, it restores the age-related decrease in the capacity to adapt to chronic stress.[522] GB has specifically been found to regulate stress-induced changes to serotonin and dopamine metabolism.[523]

GB exerts effects on several neurotransmitter systems contributing to its pharmacologic effects. Animal investigations indicate that after 14 days of administering EGb 761, there were dose-dependent increases in extracellular dopamine and acetylcholine in the medial prefrontal cortex,[524] dopamine and norepinephrine in the prefrontal cortex and to a lesser extent in the striatum,[525] and a significant decrease in norepinephrine uptake.[526] Additionally, GB extract restored 5-HT_{1A} receptor function in aged rats.[527] Bilobalide, an active constituent found in GB, was shown to increase levels of GABA and GAD (the enzyme responsible for converting glutamate to GABA) in the mouse hippocampus after four days of treatment, a finding that contributes to its anticonvulsant properties.[528] After 40 days of treatment, this same active principle increased glutamate, GABA, and glycine in the hippocampus; increased glycine in the striatum; and increased GABA in the cortex, actions that contribute to GB's broad spectrum of pharmacologic actions.[529] GB extract antagonizes cortical glycine receptors.[530] In vitro studies show that GB extract mildly blocks NMDA receptors[531] and antagonizes GABAa receptors, but not by more than 20%.[532]

Findings from animal studies give important insight into GB's effects on biological systems. In mice under various stressful conditions, it had antidepressant effects similar to those of imipramine,[533] decreased brain damage,[534] decreased anxiety-like behavior, and enhanced spatial learning and memory.[535] GB may also reduce neuron loss in mouse models of parkinsonism.[536] Given its wide-ranging pharmacologic effects and findings from animal data, GB would be expected to be beneficial in a number of medical and psychiatric conditions. There are well-designed human investigations indicating significant therapeutic effects in addressing peripheral vascular disease,[537] stroke,[538] cancer,[539] diabetic nephropathy,[540] vertigo,[541] asthma,[542] premenstrual dysphoric disorder,[543] sexual dysfunction,[544] antidepressant-induced sexual dysfunction,[545] depression-associated insomnia,[546] generalized anxiety disorder,[547] and schizophrenia.[548]

GB's ability to modulate oxidative stress, catecholamines, acetylcholine, and stress indicate that it may have cognitive enhancing effects in humans. A systematic review and meta-analysis confirm that GB extracts improve cognitive function in mild to moderate dementia,[549] but it does not appear to decrease the incidence of dementia,[550] cognitive decline, or cardiovascular events.[551] In a selective review of 29 controlled trials across various populations, GB was found to improve selective attention, long-term memory, and some aspects of executive function.[552] When the herb's effects on healthy subjects younger than 60 years were systematically reviewed, it did not have a robust effect on any aspect of cognitive functioning in short-term or long-term use.[553] However, a randomized controlled trial of EGb 761 in 66 healthy adults aged 50 to 65 years revealed a significant improvement in self-estimated mental health and quality of life.[554]

GB is not considered to be GRAS according to the FDA. It tends to be well tolerated in humans with mild side effects, including GI complaints, headache, allergic skin reactions, nausea, dizziness, restlessness, heart palpitations, and weakness.[555] EGb 761 has a half-life of four to five hours, with an absorption of at least 60%; 89% is excreted within 72 hours via exhaled carbon dioxide, urine, and feces. Oral doses in rats show sufficient concentrations of active components to exert pharmacologic effects within one or two hours.[556] In long-term (two years) toxicology and carcinogenesis studies on rodents, an extract of GB that contained 10.45 ppm of ginkgolic acid (recall that EGb 761 must contain <5 ppm) given at high doses caused an increased incidence of liver and thyroid tumors.[557]

Research on GB affecting cytochrome P450 enzymes has been contradictory and inconclusive. It is not clear whether it causes any clinically significant effect in humans.[558] There have been concerns that it may alter bleeding time and pose an increased risk of stroke; however, a systematic review and meta-analysis of the data published in 2011 concluded that there was no increased risk of bleeding associated with its use.[559] Nonetheless, it is not recommended for use with warfarin,[560] other anticoagulants, or within two weeks of surgery.[561] Caution is advised during pregnancy, especially during delivery when antiplatelet properties could increase bleeding time.[562] Use during lactation should be avoided until study results are available.[563] Secondary to data extrapolated from animal data, caution is advised in elderly populations with hypertension, as GB may impair peripheral circulation because of bradycardia and impaired hepatic function.[564] In mice, EGb 761 may increase the cataleptic effect of haloperidol when taken together,[565] and caution is advised.

A case of GB likely causing a ventricular arrhythmia on an electrocardiogram has been reported in the literature.[566] GB appears to have hormonal and endocrine effects and may influence sexual behavior, at least in a time-limited way. In vitro, GB increased the amount of testosterone produced by rat Leydig cells.[567] In rats, EGb 761 administered for 14 days caused increases in erections,[568] copulation frequency, serum testosterone levels, and sperm number and decreased serum prolactin levels.[569] These findings are thought to be related to the herb's ability to increase dopaminergic activity in certain areas of the brain.[570]

It is noteworthy that after 28 days of treatment, these effects were no longer observed, except for the increased dopamine and decreased prolactin levels.[571] In rats with impaired testicular function because of diabetes, GB extract for 12 weeks increased LH and testosterone.[572] In an open-label trial in 11 healthy volunteers (six men and five women), GB extract 240mg per day for 14 days had no effect on cortisol, 11-deoxycortisol, 17-alpha hydroxyprogesterone, testosterone, dihydrotestosterone, dehydroepiandrosterone sulfate, sex hormone-binding globulin, androstenedione, or free testosterone.[573]

Evidence for the Efficacy of Ginkgo Biloba in the Treatment of ADHD

In an open-label study, six 17- to 19-year-olds with ADHD and comorbid oppositional defiant disorder (n=3), conduct disorder (n=1), and learning disabilities (n=1) were given EGb 761 200mg per day for four weeks.[574] No other medications were allowed. The authors reported significant improvements in fidgetiness, restlessness, disruptive sounds, frustration levels, anxiety, inattention, and lack of cooperation and finishing tasks, as well as significant improvements on the 60-item Wender Utah Questionnaire. Side effects reported were stomachache and headache in two of the subjects for the first two weeks. The symptoms disappeared in one subject and remained mild in another.

In a randomized controlled trial, 50 six- to 14-year-olds with newly diagnosed ADHD combined type were given a ginkgo extract (Ginko T.D.) 80 to 120mg per day weight based or methylphenidate 20 to 30mg per day weight based for six weeks.[575] On the parent ADHD rating scale, 32% in the GB group were responders (defined as at least a 40% decrease in scores) versus 88% in the methylphenidate group. There were no significant changes on the teacher ADHD rating scale in the GB group. Limitations of this study include the use of a GB extract that did not disclose percentages of active ingredients and lack of a placebo arm for comparison.

How to Prescribe Ginkgo Biloba for ADHD

GB extract in the form of EGb 761 or other extract that is independently monitored for potency and purity may be used in adults with ADHD at doses ranging from 80 to 240mg per day divided into two or three doses daily. Because of concerns over hormonal effects, GB may be seen as conservatively contraindicated in children or may be used with caution at doses ranging from 80 to 120mg or more. Monitoring of serum testosterone and liver function may be advised in both children and adult populations. Because GB protects neuronal membranes from oxidative stress and increases EPA levels within the membrane; total antioxidant status; and levels of dopamine, norepinephrine, and acetylcholine in key brain regions, it is theoretically useful for the treatment of ADHD.

Some preliminary evidence indicates this is the case, but more well-designed studies are needed. When given with stimulants and other dopaminergic medications or supplements, GB could have additive effects. Caution is advised. Long-term high-dose use is not advised until further safety data are available. Side effects may include GI complaints, headache, allergic skin reactions, nausea, dizziness, and restlessness. Do not coadminister with anticoagulants or within two weeks of surgery or during pregnancy, labor, or lactation.

Compound Herbal Preparation

Compound herbal preparation at a glance:

May address: ADHD symptoms as assessed by the Test of Variables of Attention (TOVA)

Dose: 3mL three times daily—chamomile and passionflower were administered only to children with hyperactivity as part of their diagnosis

Time to onset of action: 4 months

AEs: None reported in this single study

GRAS: Yes, spirulina, lemon balm, chamomile, and passion-flower only

Possible MOA: Multiple—see individual herbs

Compound herbal preparation consists of *Paeoniae alba* (white peony), *Withania somnifera* (ashwagandha), *Centella asiatica* (gotu kola), *Spirulina platensis*, *Bacopa monnieri*, *Melissa officinalis* (lemon balm), chamomile, and *Passiflora incarnata* (passionflower).

Evidence for the Efficacy of Compound Herbal Preparation in the Treatment of ADHD

In a randomized controlled trial, 120 six- to 12-year-old children with DSM-IV ADHD were given 3mL of an alcohol extract tincture of these herbs three times daily for four months.[576] There were 80 children in the experimental group and 20 in the control group. Only participants with hyperactivity as part of their ADHD diagnoses were given the version of the formula that included chamomile and passionflower.

There were no serious adverse events. Results were assessed via a TOVA. There were highly significant improvements in all four dimensions of the TOVA ($p<0.0001$) for all three subtypes of ADHD. No significant improvements were found in the control group. No serious adverse events were reported, and even mild, transient complaints did not last longer than the initial two weeks of treatment and were fewer than in the placebo group. Additionally, there were no significant changes in vital signs and laboratory test values (specific laboratory test values that were monitored were not disclosed). The authors did not specify whether the extracts were standardized to specific percentages of active ingredients or what the ratios were of the herbs used in the combination formula. Considering each of these herbs separately with regard to safety and possible mechanism of action is essential before making informed prescribing decisions.

How to Prescribe Compound Herbal Preparation for ADHD
Although preliminary evidence indicates this mixture of herbs
has efficacy in ADHD, several of them may up- or downregulate
neuroendocrine and hormonal systems, which could adversely
affect development in pediatric populations. It's possible that
these contradictory effects could cancel each other out or that
the doses of each individual herb are not great enough to make
a detectable effect. Additional studies on these herbs individually and collectively are necessary to determine safety. This
compound herbal preparation may still be prescribed for ADHD
while monitoring appropriate laboratory test results, including
testosterone, LH, follicle-stimulating hormone (FSH), prolactin,
and thyroid.

Paeoniae Alba (White Peony)
White peony at a glance:

May address: No evidence of efficacy in treating ADHD as an
individual agent

Dose: Unknown

Time to onset of action: Unknown

AEs: Possible hormonal effects (see full details in the text)

GRAS: No

Possible MOA: IIO axis, cholinergic, noradrenergic

White peony is an herb that has been used for thousands of
years to treat wounds, fungal infections, pain, spasmodic
conditions,[577] and neurodegenerative disorders, including
Alzheimer's and Parkinson's disease.[578] It may have antioxidant, immunomodulating,[579] and anti-inflammatory[580] actions.
Studies show that it crosses the blood-brain barrier, has neuroprotective actions, and promotes nerve growth[581] and regeneration.[582] Animal data suggest that peony increases the levels of
serotonin in the hippocampus,[583] decreases corticosterone and

ACTH under stress,[584] and exhibits antidepressant effects.[585]

Its putative efficacy in the treatment of ADHD could be due to its ability to stimulate the release of norepinephrine,[586] its cholinergic properties,[587] and its ability to protect against glutamate-induced neurotoxicity,[588] which may be associated with ADHD. Although peony does not have GRAS status,[589] tests show that it has no obvious toxicity,[590] and it may be antimutagenic.[591] Its administration is not associated with adverse events other than gastric upset.[592] Safety during pregnancy and lactation[593] is undetermined and use should be avoided.

Peony may have anticoagulant and antiplatelet effects, leading to slowed blood clotting, potentiation of anticoagulant medications, and an increased risk of bleeding in certain populations.[594] Therefore, it should be avoided for two weeks before any surgeries. As it may require activation by intestinal flora,[595] coadministration with or after antibiotics may decrease efficacy, and consumption with probiotics could increase efficacy. It is possibly safe for short-term use up to four weeks,[596] with the most common doses being between 1.5 to 4g divided three times per day.

Prescribing Considerations for White Peony for ADHD

Peony root and less commonly flowers and stems are used medicinally. Peony tea is widely available; however, the study on ADHD above specifically used an alcohol extract. On the basis of available information, starting with a low dose of liquid extract and titrating slowly would be a conservative approach. Its likely mechanisms of action suggest that it may be best to dose peony in the morning and possibly midday but to avoid dosing late in the day, as it may be activating.

Its ability to increase norepinephrine could potentiate the effects of stimulant medications that may be prescribed. Caution is advised. As is the case with several of the herbs reviewed, peony may have hormonal effects. In vitro research indicates that it dose dependently decreases the production of testosterone in ovarian tissue.[597] Therefore, it may be conservatively contraindicated, or testosterone levels could be monitored.

Withania Somnifera (Ashwagandha)
Ashwagandha at a glance:

May address: No evidence of efficacy in treating ADHD as an individual agent

Dose: Unknown

Time to onset of action: Unknown

AEs: Possible neuroendocrine and hormonal effects (see full details in the text)

GRAS: No

Possible MOA: IIO axis, cholinergic, dopaminergic, GABAergic, serotonergic

Ashwagandha, an Ayurvedic herb that has been commonly used for more than 3000 years, has active ingredients known as *withanolides*.[598] In recent years, both animal and human research has been accumulating regarding its effects. It has antioxidant, anti-inflammatory, and immunomodulating properties.[599] It may be effective in reversing or mitigating the effects of chronic stress,[600] including lowering corticosterone and cortisol levels,[601] occurrence of ulcers, sexual dysfunction, cognitive deficits, immunosuppression, and depression.[602]

Studies suggest that because of its broad-based effects, it has a number of potential medical and psychiatric uses, including antiaging,[603] cancer treatment,[604] neurodegenerative disorders,[605] infertility, [606] anxiety,[607] depression,[608] insomnia,[609] tardive dyskinesia,[610] substance withdrawal,[611] and improving cognitive performance.[612] Specific actions on neurotransmitter systems include serotonergic,[613] dopaminergic,[614] and GABAmimetic activities,[615] as well as inhibition of acetylcholinesterase, leading to increased levels of acetylcholine,[616] which may be related to its putative cognitive enhancing properties.[617]

It is important to note that ashwagandha's effects on infertility, which include increasing testicular size,[618] initiating spermatogenesis,[619] and folliculogenesis[620] in immature rats, and improving semen concentration and motility[621] appear to be mediated by hormonal changes including increasing testosterone and LH,[622] decreasing FSH[623] and prolactin,[624] and/or possessing testosterone-like actions.[625] As these hormonal effects could have adverse effects on sexual development, this herb may be seen as conservatively contraindicated in children and adolescents. There are insufficient data at this time to determine whether and how withanolides affect developing systems of the human body. If prescribed to a pediatric population, it would be prudent to monitor testosterone and LH levels, although this would not necessarily alert practitioners to direct testosterone-like actions, if present. It may be appropriate to prescribe for adults for limited periods of time.

On the basis of its antioxidant properties and effects on acetylcholine and dopamine, it may have value in the treatment of ADHD. Although several sources state that withania extract does have GRAS status, direct FDA sources do not corroborate this claim. There are limited data with regard to pharmacodynamics. The most common adverse events include sedation[626] (likely secondary to its GABAergic actions), gastrointestinal upset, nausea, and vomiting[627] at high doses. It may potentiate the effects of other CNS depressants and sedatives.[628] Additionally, ashwagandha is reported to have thyrotropic (thyroid stimulating) effects,[629] and there is a case report of thyrotoxicosis in a 32-year-old woman.[630]

Prescribing Considerations for Ashwagandha for ADHD

Although a significant amount animal and human research is available, little is known about the pharmacodynamic param-

eters, safety, and toxicity of ashwagandha. This makes it difficult to apply a medical model to its administration. It is widely
available from a number of manufacturers in extract and raw
forms. Doses may range from 300 to 500mg per day of extract
commonly standardized to 1.5% withanolides, 6 to 12ml per
day of 1:2 fluid extract, or up to 3 to 6g per day of dried root.[631]
Sedation is a common adverse effect, and evening dosing is
often recommended.

Ashwagandha is conservatively contraindicated in children
because of its gonadotropic and possibly thyrotropic effects. If
it is prescribed, it would be prudent to monitor testosterone and
LH levels at baseline and during treatment. Administration to
adults may be appropriate, but, as with many herbs, use should
be limited to several weeks before taking at least two weeks
off. It should be avoided during pregnancy and breastfeeding.
Use caution when CNS depressants and thyroid conditions are
present. It may make sense to monitor thyroid parameters.

Centella Asiatica (Gotu Kola)
Gotu kola at a glance:

May address: No evidence of efficacy in treating ADHD as an
individual agent

Dose: Unknown

Time to onset of action: Unknown

AEs: Possible neuroendocrine and hormonal effects (see full
details in the text)

GRAS: No

Possible MOA: IIO axis, cholinergic, dopaminergic, noradrenergic, GABAergic, serotonergic

Gotu kola is an herb that has been used for thousands of years
in Asian medicine.[632] It has notable antioxidant, anti-inflamma-

tory, and immunomodulating actions.[633] Evidence suggests that it has a number of medicinal uses, including wound healing,[634] venous insufficiency,[635] diabetes,[636] epilepsy,[637] inflammatory bowel disease,[638] scleroderma,[639] and several forms of cancer.[640] It possesses actions within the central nervous system that could make it a viable treatment for ADHD as well as for other psychiatric disorders. Studies show that it modulates the activity of acetylcholinesterase.

Depending on the situation, it may increase[641] or decrease[642] the activity of this enzyme, resulting in subsequent changes to levels of acetylcholine (Ach). It also increases levels of serotonin, dopamine, and norepinephrine,[643] as well as GAD activity,[644] the enzyme that metabolizes glutamate to GABA, which may account for the observed increased levels of the latter.[645] It decreases levels of corticosterone under stressful conditions and protects against glutamate-induced neurotoxicity.[646] It is neuroprotective against a variety of toxic substances.[647] Therefore, it may have efficacy in treating depression,[648] anxiety,[649] age-related memory decline,[650] Alzheimer's dementia,[651] and ADHD.[652] It appears to have cognitive enhancing effects,[653] improving learning and memory.[654]

As is the case with a number of herbs, animal data indicate that it has hormonal and fertility effects, including decreased sperm count, motility, viability, spermatogenic cells, testosterone, FSH, and LH, making gotu kola a potential antifertility and anti-spermatogenic agent.[655] Until further data are available documenting the hormonal effects in humans, it should conservatively be avoided in children and some populations of adult clients. If it is prescribed, it would be reasonable to monitor testosterone, FSH, and LH levels.

Prescribing Considerations for Gotu Kola for ADHD

Although the amount of animal and human research is growing, and this herb may have therapeutic effects for a number of medical and psychiatric disorders, information regarding safety, hormonal effects, and pharmacodynamics is limited. It is not considered GRAS according to the FDA and is conservatively contraindicated in children because of its antifertility and antispermatogenic effects. If it is prescribed, it would be prudent to monitor testosterone, FSH, and LH levels at baseline and during treatment.

It may be used with caution for limited periods in some adults with ADHD. Prescribing concerns include hormonal and antifertility action,[656] effects on cytochrome P450 enzymes (inhibits CYP2C9 and others),[657] and the possibility of decreased metabolism and toxicity at high, long-term doses.[658] There also are three case studies of reversible jaundice.[659] It should be avoided during pregnancy owing to the risk of spontaneous abortion.[660] No safety information is available with regard to breastfeeding. The most common adverse events are GI upset, nausea, and rash (when used topically).[661] Common doses of the extract range from 60 to 120mg per day.[662] Use for more than six weeks is not recommended without taking a break of at least two weeks.[663]

Spirulina Platensis
Spirulina at a glance:

May address: Inattention, hyperactivity, impulsivity (when considered as a form of multinutrient therapy), and allergic rhinitis

Dose: 250mg to several grams per day

Time to onset of action: Unknown, possibly weeks to months

AEs: GI upset (see full details in the text)

GRAS: Yes (considered safe even for infants and young children)

Possible MOA when considered as a form of multinutrient therapy: IIO axis, neurotransmitter synthesis, membrane-lipid therapy

Spirulina platensis is a well-studied microscopic filamentous alga with a long history of human use as a food and a food supplement.[664] It has documented antioxidant, anti-inflammatory, and immunoenhancing properties and may be useful in diabetes, dyslipidemia, cancer, and viral and bacterial infections.[665] As a food, it is quite nutritionally dense,[666] providing protein, essential fats, and a wide array of vitamins and minerals, including beta-carotene, B vitamins, vitamin C, iron, magnesium, and zinc. Spirulina also increases the absorption of vitamin B1 and other vitamins and acts as a prebiotic, providing nutrition to beneficial microorganisms in the gut.[667] Accordingly, it may be thought of as a multinutrient approach to treating ADHD and other psychiatric disorders.

Animal studies indicate that it may have potential applications in psychiatry as an antidepressant,[668] a preventive agent for haloperidol-induced tardive dyskinesia,[669] and a means to prevent neurodegenerative changes and age-related decline in noradrenergic receptor function.[670] However, apart from the study cited above, the literature does not support its use as a treatment for ADHD, unless the issue of allergic rhinitis is taken into account. In animal studies, spirulina prevents the release of histamine from mast cells[671] and dose dependently inhibits allergic responses.[672]

In randomized controlled trials in adults with allergic rhinitis, it decreased the inflammatory mediator interleukin 4 by 32% at a dose of 2g per day over a 12-week period[673] and significantly improved symptoms and physical findings (p<0.001), including nasal discharge, sneezing, nasal congestion, and itching.[674] Hence, its application to ADHD may be expanded to include this common comorbid condition.

Prescribing Considerations for *Spirulina Platensis* for ADHD
Spirulina has GRAS status granted by the FDA and is considered to be safe for daily consumption even for infants and young children on the basis of extensive animal and human toxicology

tests.[675] It has been used as a dietary supplement in malnourished children and adults with positive effects.[676] As a multinutrient approach to treating ADHD and to target comorbid symptoms of allergic rhinitis, spirulina may be given at doses ranging from 250mg to several grams per day. Caution is advised when using it in patients who use anticoagulants because of high levels of vitamin K, which may interfere with the action of these medications. Similarly, caution is advised in patients using immunosuppressants.

Bacopa Monnieri
Bacopa at a glance:

May address: Cognitive performance in the setting of ADHD in children

Dose: 100mg per day of extract

Time to onset of action: 12 weeks

AEs: Antifertility and antispermatogenic effects (see full details in the text)

GRAS: No

Possible MOA: IIO axis, cholinergic, modulates glutamate, serotonergic

Bacopa monnieri is another antioxidant, anti-inflammatory Ayurvedic herb traditionally used as a brain tonic to enhance memory, learning, and concentration.[677] It may have medical applications for epilepsy, cancer, asthma, bronchitis, and gastric ulcers.[678] Several actions within the central nervous system may make it a viable treatment for some psychiatric conditions.

Animal data indicate that bacopa inhibits acetylcholinesterase[679] in a way that is similar to that of donepezil[680] and decreases dopamine[681] and stress-induced corticosterone levels.[682] It increases 5-HT(3A) receptor (a type of serotonin receptor) expression[683] and mRNA of serotonin-synthesizing enzymes[684] and serotonin[685] (although another study[686] found decreased serotonin and increased dopamine levels). It also protects against glutamate excitotoxicity[687] and GABA receptor downregulation[688] in the setting of epilepsy and reversed benzodiazepine-induced amnesia.[689]

Given these possible mechanisms of action, this herb may improve symptoms of ADHD,[690] be beneficial to learning and memory,[691] have antianxiety effects[692] comparable to those of lorazepam,[693] and have antidepressant effects[694] similar to those of imipramine.[695] It appears that long-term administration (12 weeks) is required for cognitive enhancing effects.[696] In a randomized controlled trial that was published as an abstract only,[697] bacopa extract at 100mg per day for 12 weeks in 19 children with DSM-IV ADHD significantly improved sentence repetition, logical memory, and paired associate learning without any significant adverse events. These effects were maintained through 16 weeks, after four weeks of placebo administration. Another study involving 28 children with IQs between 70 and 90 who received bacopa extract at 225mg per day for four months observed significant improvements in working memory and short-term memory without major adverse events.[698]

In a review of randomized controlled trials on bacopa as a cognitive enhancer from 2012, it was found to improve memory and free recall in healthy, nondemented subjects and subjects with memory complaints but no major cognitive impairment.[699] Doses used were in the range of 300 to 450mg per day for three months. However, a more recent study published in January 2013 found no significant change in cognitive performance in 72 healthy adults receiving bacopa extract 450mg per day for 12 weeks.[700] A trend toward decreased anxiety was noted.

Once again, this is an herb with apparent antifertility and antispermatogenic effects.[701] Mice receiving bacopa for 28 to

56 days had decreased sperm motility, viability, and number of sperm in the epididymis, as well as alterations in the seminiferous tubules. There was no effect on testosterone or libido, but fertility was suppressed. These findings were reversible within 56 days after treatment. Further studies on spermatogenic effects in humans are required prior to bacopa being medically endorsed. Although this herb looks like a promising treatment for ADHD and other cognitive issues, the long-term treatment requirement and fertility ramifications make it conservatively contraindicated.

Prescribing Considerations for *Bacopa Monnieri* for ADHD

Bacopa does not have GRAS status. Apart from antifertility concerns in males, making it conservatively contraindicated in children until more safety data are available, high doses in mice have increased the thyroid hormone T4 by 41%.[702] Use caution in thyroid disorders. It has a mild sedative effect[703] and may potentiate other central nervous system sedatives. Otherwise, in human[704] and animal[705] safety data, it appears to be nontoxic. Gastrointestinal upset is a common side effect.[706] Doses range from 5 to 10g per day of raw herb powder, 200 to 400mg per day of extract standardized to 2% bacosides, and 100 to 200mg per day in children.[707]

Melissa Officinalis (Lemon Balm)

Lemon balm at a glance:

May address: No evidence of efficacy in treating ADHD as an individual agent

Dose: Unknown

AEs: Possibly sedating, possible interaction with thyroid medications (see full details in the text)

Time to onset of action: Unknown

GRAS: Yes

Possible MOA: Antioxidant, cholinergic, GABAergic

Lemon balm is a member of the mint family that has been used for centuries for anxiety, insomnia, low appetite, pain, indigestion,[708] nervous tension, depression, and epilepsy.[709] Animal research indicates that it may be effective for diabetes,[710] inflammatory pain,[711] and cancer,[712] and it may have antiviral[713] and antimicrobial[714] properties. As is the case with a number of other herbs, it decreases corticosterone[715] levels and is a powerful antioxidant,[716] especially with regard to lipid peroxidation.[717] In humans, it protects against radiation-induced DNA damage.[718]

Animal and human studies report that lemon balm may have antianxiety,[719] sleep-improving,[720] and cognitive enhancing effects.[721] These findings may be related to inhibition of GABA transaminase[722] (the enzyme that metabolizes and deactivates the neurotransmitter GABA) and cholinergic agonism at the receptor site level.[723] Although the GABAergic action tends to lower anxiety, higher doses may be associated with sedation and decreased alertness. Therefore, care must be taken when titrating the dose.

When used in combination with another herb called *valerian*, lemon balm may improve symptoms associated with ADHD. In an open-label trial in 918 children younger than 12 years with restlessness and dyssomnias who were given the combination of herbs for four weeks, there were significant improvements (p value not reported) in symptoms, with good tolerability and no adverse events deemed to be related to the intervention.[724]

Prescribing Considerations for Lemon Balm for ADHD
Lemon balm is considered to be GRAS according to the FDA[725] and appears to be safe for administration to adults and children. It should not be used during pregnancy or breastfeeding.[726] It may potentiate the effects of sedative medications and may interact with thyroid medications.[727] In safety studies, it has

antigenotoxic and antimutagenic properties (prevents DNA damage).[728]

In psychiatry, its main application is for anxiety disorders, but it may possibly be effective for hyperactivity, restlessness, and insomnia associated with ADHD. Commonly used doses of lemon balm extract in adults are 300 to 600mg per day and in children are 75 to 300mg per day.

Chamomile
Chamomile at a glance:

May address: Inattention, hyperactivity, impulsivity

May allow for lower dose of stimulant medication when used adjunctively

May protect against tics associated with stimulant medication

Dose: 100mg extract and 190mg of essential oil per day

Time to onset of action: 4 weeks

AEs: Sedation, allergic reactions, possible antithymus activity at high doses for long periods (see full details in the text)

GRAS: Yes

Possible MOA: IIO axis, dopaminergic, noradrenergic, glutamate modulation, GABAergic

Chamomile (*Matricaria chamomilla*) is one of the most commonly used herbs in the world with a long history of human consumption. Traditional uses include colic, bloating, upper respiratory infections, menstrual pain, anxiety, insomnia, hay fever, inflammation, muscle spasms, menstrual disorders, insomnia, ulcers, wounds, gastrointestinal disorders, rheumatic pain, and hemorrhoids.[729] It has known antimicrobial,[730] antioxidant,[731] anti-inflammatory,[732] immunomodulating,[733] and anticancer[734] properties. Chamomile has multiple active constituents, which vary depending upon how the herb is processed. Water and alcohol extracts contain the main active ingredient, apigenin, and the essential oil of chamomile contains higher levels of alpha-bisabolol and bisabolol oxide A. There are numerous studies on the effects of chamomile and its active ingredients, which often provide conflicting evidence, depending upon how the herb was processed and whether the investigations were in vitro or in vivo.

In vitro, water and alcohol chamomile extracts were found to inhibit the activity of the enzyme glutamate decarboxylase (GAD), which converts glutamate to GABA.[735] This suggests that chamomile would lead to excitation of the central nervous system secondary to lowered levels of the inhibitory neurotransmitter GABA. The authors conclude that this inhibitory effect on GABA must be confirmed in vivo because certain phytochemicals can be metabolized or have limited bioavailability in the brain. An in vivo animal study on the effects of apigenin reported increased activity of GAD along with prolongation of sleep time induced by the medication phenobarbital, which is a GABAa agonist.[736]

The in vivo findings support the use of this particular component of chamomile as an anxiolytic and sedative agent. In animals, apigenin has been found to decrease locomotor activity,[737] decrease anxiety, and have affinity for the central benzodiazepine receptor.[738] Conversely, animal data have shown that apigenin does not decrease anxiety[739] and is not counteracted by flumazenil, a medication that inhibits the binding of benzodiazepines to the GABAa receptor.[740] An in vitro study on the effects of apigenin reports that, at high doses, it antagonizes GABAa receptors, but at low doses, it enhances the effect of diazepam (a benzodiazepine) on GABA receptors.[741] The authors conclude that apigenin's effects on GABA receptors are complex. In rats under stress, apigenin acts as an antidepressant like the medication fluoxetine, decreases levels of corticosterone, and attenuates stress-induced changes to the neurotransmitters serotonin and dopamine in several brain regions.[742]

It also functions as a monoamine transporter, possibly affecting levels of dopamine and norepinephrine.[743] It has antidepressant effects in mice at lower doses that may be mediated by dopaminergic mechanisms (as the effects were blocked by haloperidol, a D2 receptor antagonist), but at higher doses, this antidepressant effect was lost.[744] Studies also indicate that apigenin acts as an MAO inhibitor,[745] potentially affecting the metabolism of several neurotransmitters. Without evidence to the contrary, apigenin inhibits glutamate-induced calcium signaling by blocking NMDA,[746] AMPA, and metabotropic glutamate receptors.[747] It also blocks voltage-gated calcium channels and caffeine-induced calcium release.[748] This indicates that apigenin may provide neuroprotection against glutamate-induced neurotoxicity,[749] and this overall reduction of neural network excitability may account for its sedative effects,[750] as opposed to or in addition to a GABAergic mechanism.

The essential oil of chamomile, with high levels of alpha-bisabolol, has been found to exert anxiogenic (anxiety producing) effects similar to the stimulant caffeine.[751] Not surprisingly, when the essential oil of chamomile was studied as an intervention for primary insomnia in adult humans in a randomized controlled trial, it was not found to be effective.[752] However, in sleep-disturbed rats, the water extract of chamomile significantly decreased sleep latency, which was antagonized by flumazenil.[753] The authors concluded that the sleep-promoting/hypnotic effects of chamomile are benzodiazepine-like and may be due to effects on benzodiazepine receptors.

When assessing the usefulness of this or any herb, it is important to examine well-designed controlled trials. Controlled human trials give preliminary evidence that chamomile extracts standardized to 1.2% apigenin are well tolerated and effective for mild to moderate generalized anxiety disorder[754] and depression[755] when administered over an eight-week period. Evidence that chamomile as monotherapy is effective for ADHD is limited to one small placebo-controlled observational study. Two patients, one 14 years old and one 16 years old, with ADHD inattentive subtype were given 100mg of chamomile extract along with 190mg of essential oil three times per day for four weeks.[756] Both were previously using methylphenidate for six years but had the common side effects of insomnia and weight loss. On the ADHD rating scale (ADHD RS), according to children, parents, and teachers, inattention decreased from a score of 14 to 9, hyperactivity/impulsivity decreased from 13 to 7, and the total score decreased from 27 to 16.

On the Clinical Global Impression (CGI) scale, a blinded physician rated the subjects as being much improved. However, no significant improvement was seen on the Conners' Continuous Performance Test. There were no serious side effects and no significant changes in laboratory test or electrocardiographic results. Mild transitory sedation was reported. The authors concluded that chamomile used adjunctively could permit a lower dose of stimulant medication and may provide protection against tics.

Chamomile is GRAS according to the FDA[757] and tends to be well tolerated with few adverse events. However, an in vitro study found that bisabolol oxide A, which is found in chamomile, caused apoptosis (cell death) in rat thymocytes (normal noncancerous thymus cells).[758] This was observed to occur at higher micromolar concentrations of 30 to 100 when incubated with these cells for 24 hours. This did not occur when the concentration was 10 micromolar or less, nor did it occur with high concentrations over shorter periods of time (three hours as opposed to 24 hours). To put this in perspective, the amount of bisabolol oxide A is calculated to be approximately 300mg in 100g of dry flowers. If one uses 1 to 3g of chamomile to make a cup of tea, then the amount of bisabolol oxide A per cup is 3 to 9mg, which is 12.5 to 37.5 micromolar.[759]

Therefore, when chamomile is used conventionally, it is unlikely to be cytotoxic to our normal thymus cells. However, dosing strategies designed to maintain high serum levels of chamomile's active components (including bisabolol oxide A) over long periods could theoretically result in cytotoxicity to thymus or other cells in the body. Until safety studies are performed in this regard, chamomile used in this manner is conservatively contraindicated. Its conventional use periodically as tea appears to be safe.

Prescribing Considerations for Chamomile for ADHD
Because of concerns over potential cytotoxicity to thymus and possibly other cells, chamomile should not be used at high doses multiple times per day over long periods until safety studies have been performed. Chamomile is GRAS according to the FDA. It should not be given in large amounts during pregnancy, as it may induce uterine contractions. Caution should be used in clients who are allergic to ragweed or daisies (chamomile is a member of this family). Constituents in the herb may interfere with blood clotting, and its use should be avoided when aspirin, warfarin, and other anticoagulants are being used. Chamomile could potentiate the effects of benzodiazepines and other sedative medications.[760] When used periodically in the form of tea or extract, it appears to be a safe and possibly effective treatment for occasional anxiety and insomnia.

Passiflora Incarnata (Passionflower)
Passionflower at a glance:

May address: No evidence of efficacy in treating ADHD as an individual agent

Dose: Unknown

Time to onset of action: Unknown

AEs: Possible antithyroid activity, potential toxicity of some constituents, sedation (see full details in the text)

GRAS: Yes

Possible MOA: IIO axis, cholinergic, dopaminergic, noradrenergic, GABAergic, serotonergic

Passiflora is a genus of herbs with hundreds of species that are native to the Western hemisphere.[761] Indigenous North Americans historically used it as a sedative.[762] It has also been used as a hypnotic agent and for nervous gastrointestinal complaints.[763] Passionflower was approved for "nervous unrest" in Germany in 1985[764] and is considered GRAS according to the FDA.[765] Several species have been studied for medicinal value, but *Passiflora incarnata* (PI) has been more extensively investigated and is the most widely available.

PI is an herb with complex actions owing to the presence of several known active constituents, including vitexin, isovitexin, chrysin, and harmane. It is commonly standardized to a certain percentage of vitexin or isovitexin, although other components are still present. Therefore, it is necessary to examine research on PI as a whole herb and its proposed active ingredients independently.

PI extract is an antioxidant[766] that may have medicinal uses for diabetes, hyperlipidemia,[767] asthma,[768] and nicotine dependence[769] and may act as an antitussive similarly to codeine.[770] It appears to be GABAergic, interacting with the GABA site of the GABAa receptor.[771] Its actions have been reported to be blocked by flumazenil, a benzodiazepine receptor site antagonist.[772] It may also interact with the opioid system as evidenced by its antitussive action[773] and antagonism by naloxone, an opioid receptor antagonist.[774]

In animal studies, PI extract has been repeatedly found to act as an anxiolytic (in one study comparable with diazepam),[775]

sedative,[776] and antiseizure agent.[777] However, it was found to be anxiogenic when given to mice in their drinking water. The authors suggested that the herb may have both anxiolytic and anxiogenic properties at different doses, with increased anxiety at high doses.[778] Another study found that it decreases anxiety only at certain doses; if dosed too high or too low, anxiolysis was not observed.[779] In mice, the herb was found to be an aphrodisiac, resulting in significantly increased mounting behavior at certain doses.[780] Additional studies are needed to determine the mechanism of action of this effect, as it could represent a contraindication in certain populations. Controlled human trials indicate that PI extract decreases anxiety prior to surgery[781] and is as effective as oxazepam (a benzodiazepine medication) for the treatment of generalized anxiety disorder.[782] PI in the form of tea in healthy subjects improved subjective sleep quality.[783] In opiate-addicted patients, PI added to clonidine was effective in addressing the mental symptoms associated with opiate withdrawal.[784] There is no direct evidence that PI has therapeutic efficacy for ADHD as monotherapy.

Vitexin is a constituent of PI for which the extract may be standardized. It has antioxidant,[785] anti-inflammatory,[786] anti-cancer,[787] and cardioprotective properties.[788] Animal studies indicate that it may regulate pain sensation via interaction with opioid receptors[789] and be an anticonvulsant via its actions at the benzodiazepine site of the GABAa receptor.[790] In mice, it exerts an antidepressant effect mediated by an increase in catecholamines (norepinephrine and dopamine) in the synaptic cleft and interactions with 5-HT1A, alpha-2, and dopamine receptors.[791] In rats, it may play a role in memory function via modulation of cholinergic receptors.[792]

Taken together, these actions in the central nervous system could theoretically translate to efficacy in the treatment of ADHD, as well as other psychiatric conditions, including anxiety, depression, and dementia. Additional studies are required to determine whether this is the case in humans. Vitexin, however, has documented antithyroid activity[793] secondary to its ability to inhibit the enzyme thyroid peroxidase.[794] This finding suggests that patients taking PI should be monitored for hypothyroidism, and its use may be contraindicated in certain populations.

Another active constituent of PI is isovitexin.[795] Research suggests that it has antioxidant,[796] immunomodulating,[797] and antidiabetic[798] actions and appears to be nontoxic at high doses.[799] There is no evidence in the literature with regard to its application for psychiatric disorders as monotherapy.

Chrysin, also found in PI, is an antioxidant,[800] immunomodulator,[801] and anticonvulsant[802] and may have applications in the treatment[803] and prevention[804] of cancer. Like whole PI herb, chrysin interacts with the GABAa receptor,[805] possibly being a partial agonist at the benzodiazepine receptor,[806] and its actions are antagonized by flumazenil.[807] In animal studies, it acts as an anxiolytic comparable with the benzodiazepines midazolam[808] and diazepam.[809] However, it has been found to be toxic to trout liver cells because they express myeloperoxidase, an enzyme that is also expressed in a subtype of human white blood cells.[810] Therefore, the safety of high doses over time is questionable. This potential risk may be mitigated by the fact that chrysin has poor oral bioavailability,[811] a finding that could also call into question its therapeutic effects. Additional information in the form of controlled human trials is needed.

Harmane, another molecule found in PI, is a naturally occurring antioxidant[812] found in the mammalian central nervous system[813] that protects against lipid peroxidation.[814] As is the case with other active compounds in PI, it has GABA-potentiating properties.[815] Harmane is also a reversible MAO inhibitor[816] and has anxiolytic and antidepressant effects[817] observed in animal research. At low doses, it is an anticonvulsant, but at high doses it tends to increase seizures.[818] Harmane has been described as a tremor-inducing toxin, which is found to be elevated in patients who have tremors.[819] Ingestion of harmane in humans has toxic effects, including hallucination, excitation, elation, and euphoria, and at high doses can cause tremors and convulsions.[820] It increases plasma ACTH, corticosterone, serotonin, and norepinephrine.[821]

Certain doses can impair learning and working memory.[822] It also serves a neuromodulatory role in the forebrain reward system.[823] In summary, this component of PI is an endogenous antioxidant that has several potentially therapeutic and toxic effects. The concentration of harmane in PI is not generally standardized, so it is difficult to determine the amount that is ingested when consuming PI extract.

PI is an herb that has GRAS status according to the FDA. It is generally considered safe by experts, with few adverse events when used as a food additive and taken by healthy individuals in recommended doses for short durations.[824] It does not appear to be toxic at high doses over longer periods (180 days).[825] There are insufficient data in children for a safety determination to be made. It is possibly unsafe during pregnancy and lactation because it may stimulate uterine contractions.[826] It should be avoided in very young children and those with severe liver or kidney disease.[827]

PI may potentiate the effects of central nervous system depressants, MAO inhibitors, and anticoagulant and antiplatelet medications.[828] There are case reports of hand tremors, dizziness, and muscle fatigue when PI is mixed with valerian root and benzodiazepine,[829] as well as severe nausea, vomiting, drowsiness, and electrocardiographic changes requiring hospitalization and cardiac monitoring.[830]

Prescribing Considerations for Passionflower for ADHD
Because of concerns over *Passiflora incarnata*'s narrow therapeutic index, antithyroid activity, possible toxicity to human cells that express the enzyme myeloperoxidase, and potential toxic effects of harmane, its high-dose use for long durations

is not recommended until further safety studies are available. Once deemed to be safe, vitexin may be the component of PI that could be the most useful for ADHD symptoms. It is likely safe for short-term use as an antianxiety, sedative, hypnotic agent, as well as for the mental symptoms associated with opiate withdrawal. It is often ingested as tea made from dried leaves or as a liquid or powdered extract often standardized to certain percentages of vitexin or isovitexin.

Chapter 14

Clinical Scenarios

What follows are commonly encountered clinical situations associated with ADHD in which NBP can be applied. It is not intended to replace, but rather complement, other effective and necessary treatment modalities.

Treatment-Naïve Clients

What approach to take with previously untreated clients with a new diagnosis depends largely upon the severity of symptoms and desires of the patient. Severe symptoms associated with behavioral or academic issues that must be promptly addressed respond well to medications in most cases. In such cases, the use of FDA-approved medications for the treatment of ADHD should be discussed with parents and patients. NBP can then be implemented once a degree of symptom relief has been established. If the client wishes to avoid the use of medication, comprehensive and targeted approaches work for severe as well as milder cases. Unfortunately, NBP can take days to weeks to take effect, whereas stimulants require only hours.

Although they may be treating only part of the problem, stimulants' rapid onset, high efficacy, and ease of use make them attractive choices. When modulating dopamine and norepinephrine are needed for symptom control, these medications do it more rapidly and powerfully than natural interventions can. A targeted NBP approach, as guided by laboratory test values and specific symptoms, is preferable when compliance with complex supplement regimens is limited.

For clients responsive to prescription medication without significant adverse effects or comorbidities, the only NBP approaches suggested would be correcting for aberrant laboratory test values and a targeted approach aimed at decreasing the dose of medication, if this reflects the wishes of the client or parents. Supplements and/or dietary interventions can be implemented, with periodic trials of decreasing the medication.

Clients may be responsive to prescription medication but with significant adverse effects. Commonly observed adverse effects associated with stimulant medications include GI upset, lack of appetite, insomnia, anxiety, irritability, headaches, and affective dulling (flat affect and lack of spontaneity, creativity, and sense of humor). In some cases, decreasing the dose of medication resolves the problem(s) but can result in lack of efficacy in treating ADHD symptoms. The stepwise addition of supplements, starting with those addressing low laboratory test values (iron and zinc in particular) and progressing through other essential, metabolic, and herbal supplements, usually allows for a decreased dose of medication without sacrificing efficacy. NBP approaches can also target some of these side effects directly. For example, probiotics can help with GI upset; L-theanine, magnesium, and melatonin can be used for insomnia; lemon balm, for anxiety; zinc, for affective blunting; and ALCAR, for irritability and headaches. When NBP is used in this capacity, it also must be monitored for the incidence of side effects.

Clients may be partially responsive or unresponsive to prescription medications. Medications prescribed for ADHD do a great job at modulating the catecholamines (dopamine and norepinephrine), a strategy that is usually effective. Although NBP can address these neurotransmitter systems to a significant degree, they do not do it as powerfully and rapidly as medications can. When medicines do not work or only partially work, this may reflect the multifactorial etiology of ADHD. Targeting dysfunction in the IIO axis, neurotransmitter synthesis, membrane lipids, and other neurotransmitter systems is essential in some patients to achieve symptom control. Therefore, if medications have been partially effective, they are continued as NBP is implemented in a comprehensive or abbreviated way.

Clients with Comorbid Gastrointestinal (GI) Symptoms

GI symptoms in the setting of ADHD commonly occur for three reasons: medication or supplement adverse effect, anxiety, and food intolerance. Clues to the cause lie in the specific types of symptoms and patterns. GI upset due to medications or supplements often presents as abdominal pain or nausea occurring minutes to hours after ingestion of the offending agent. It often disappears on its own with time or if it is taken with food. When time and food do not help, the dose could be lowered or the intervention could be discontinued.

Anxiety can often present with somatic complaints that may be GI in nature and include abdominal pain, nausea, lack of appetite, diarrhea, or constipation. Anxiety-induced GI issues usually occur prior to or during anxiety-provoking situations. In children, there is often a pattern of symptoms in the morning before school or tests, whereas the symptoms are absent on weekends and holidays. Stimulants and stimulating supplements can exacerbate anxiety and consequently worsen associated GI symptoms. As a rule, it is best to address anxiety prior to treating ADHD. This can be achieved via psychotherapy, pharmacotherapy, or specific NBP protocols that will be detailed in a future volume. There are instances when anxiety is largely or partially responsible for what is presumed to be ADHD symptoms. Once anxiety is adequately treated, residual symptoms of ADHD may then be addressed. GI symptoms related to food intolerance can manifest as abdominal pain, nausea, flatulence, diarrhea, and constipation. The symptoms can occur within minutes, hours or sometimes days of eating the offending food and are absent when it is eliminated from the diet. Supplementing with probiotics can be helpful.

Clients with Comorbid Allergic Rhinitis (AR)

AR is commonly seen in the allergic/hypersensitive subtype of ADHD. The two main causes of the symptoms are seasonal allergies and food sensitivities. In either case, referral to an allergist for testing and treatment is recommended. For food-based AR, elimination diets can help determine which foods are causing the problem. Probiotics and spirulina may be effective in treating and preventing AR.

Clients with Sleep Difficulties

Sleep difficulties in the setting of ADHD are commonly due to medication and supplement side effects and anxiety. When due to the former, supplementing with L-theanine, melatonin, or magnesium may improve sleep parameters. Sometimes it is necessary to reduce or eliminate the agent that is causing the problem. When due to anxiety, sleep problems may only manifest the night before anxiety-provoking situations, such as school, work, or social and sporting events. Treatment of anxiety with psychotherapy, pharmacotherapy, or NBP may be advised prior to treating ADHD with stimulants, depending on what is the most problematic diagnosis.

Chapter 15

Treating ADHD with NBP
Phase III: Follow-Up, Monitoring, Adjustments, and Troubleshooting

In a majority of cases, implementing these treatment suggestions will result in significant improvement of ADHD symptoms. When therapeutic effects are lacking, reconsidering
dietary modifications, including elimination or restriction
diets, is advised. If stimulant medications, atomoxetine, and/
or alpha-2 agonists have not yet been considered or tried, they
are recommended as first-line FDA-approved interventions that
may be used with NBP at this juncture or during any phase of
treatment. Rechecking and correlating levels of RBC n-6:n-3
ratio, RBC magnesium, zinc, ferritin, and vitamin D with clinical
improvement (or the lack thereof) is recommended.

Follow Up, Monitor, and Adjust

1. If results are lacking, revisit dietary interventions, especially restriction diets.

2. Consider monitoring appropriate laboratory test results
   and correlate with clinical improvements.

3. Consider the use of prescription medications, including
   stimulants, atomoxetine, and/or alpha-2 agonists.

4. Adjust doses of supplements according to increases in body
   mass or age.

As is the case with many prescription medications, adjustments in doses of supplements may be necessary as body mass
increases. This is especially true for supplements with dosing
recommendations that are weight or age based like magnesium, pycnogenol, and zinc. Many clients just don't like taking
vitamins. This can be addressed by using dietary interventions

whenever possible and/or consuming certain supplements with food like juice, applesauce, yogurt, or smoothies.

Supplements that can be taken this way include theanine, melatonin, vitamin D3, probiotics, PS, zinc, and possibly pycnogenol, as these have minimal to no flavor. This approach will not work with ALCAR or NAC because they have strong bitter flavors. Fish oil can be consumed in liquid form with juice, but it tends to float on top. What seems to work better is taking a "shot" of cold fish oil with a juice "chaser." Fish oil is a supplement that does not need to be taken daily. Some clients prefer to take a tablespoon every few days instead of a teaspoon daily. When herbs are used, it is advisable to take them for a period of four to six weeks before taking at least two weeks off.

Chapter 16

In Summary

The human body is composed of highly complex systems that work in unison to allow for the functioning of the organism as a whole. The CNS (brain and spinal cord) are arguably the most intricate of these systems. A number of interdependent factors influence the functioning of our bodies, including genetic variation, presence or lack of essential materials (especially at critical periods of development), presence of toxins and antinutrients, injuries, aging, and psychosocial and environmental factors. Inevitably, in the course of living, things go awry and our bodies do not function perfectly. When a certain threshold of dysfunction is reached, this is known as disease.

When the brain is affected, psychological disease can be the result. Psychiatrists are specially trained to diagnose and treat these types of conditions. Years of intense study are required to gain a thorough understanding of the body and CNS sufficient to treat mental disorders. However, medical and psychiatric training may not emphasize the effect that nutritional factors can have on the etiology, presentation, and comorbidities associated with psychiatric conditions.

As a mainstay of current practice, medications are commonly prescribed by psychiatrists to treat mental disorders. Such medications, having profound effects on mood, behavior, and cognition, can improve the quality of lives of those suffering from mental illnesses. In some instances, however, they may have adverse effects or are only partially effective or ineffective. For various reasons, clients may wish to avoid or minimize the use of synthetic psychotropic medications. The nutrient-based approach to psychiatry is designed to be an organized, systematic, and evidence-based way to augment the biochemical approaches used in psychiatry.

The majority of psychiatric disorders are associated with oxidative stress, inflammation, immune system dysfunction, and/or membrane lipid abnormalities. These factors also underlie most medical illnesses, many of which occur comorbidly with some psychiatric conditions. The ability of nutrient-based psychiatry to regulate these key systems may be partly responsible for its therapeutic benefits, may address or prevent comorbid conditions, and may benefit the patient's overall health.

Those suffering from mental disorders who desire to avoid synthetic medications, have outstanding symptoms, and/ or experience untoward side effects resulting from standard psychiatric interventions currently have limited options. Results of the current state of affairs include lack of client compliance with medications prescribed by psychiatrists, self-medication, and clients seeking alternative providers, who may be adept but do not have the training to integrate prescription medications with nutritional interventions. This latter situation may result in fragmented and uncoordinated treatment strategies that are not optimal. It is my hope that nutrient-based psychiatry will help to educate those on both sides of the equation, patients and doctors, thereby having a significant effect on decreasing psychiatric morbidity.

Appendix

Quick-Reference Prescribing Guide for NBP Treatment of ADHD

I. Assessment

Assess for both breathing- and nonbreathing-related sleep disorders, dietary habits, and presence of food allergies. Make appropriate referrals to allergists; ear, nose, and throat specialists; and primary care physicians if breathing-related sleep disorders are present.

Laboratory tests:
1. Serum zinc

2. Ferritin

3. RBC omega-6:omega-3 ratio

4. RBC magnesium

5. 25-hydroxyvitamin D

II. Treatment

Suggested dietary modifications:

1. Increase n-3 fats and decrease n-6 fats

2. Increase magnesium and vitamin B6

3. Increase zinc

4. Increase iron (if necessary)

5. Avoid fluctuations in blood sugar and increase protein intake

6. Avoid pesticides

7. Use restriction and elimination diets

8. Address nonbreathing-related sleep disorders

L-theanine at a glance:
May address: Improves sleep parameters in the setting of ADHD

Dose: 200-500mg 1 hour prior to bedtime

Time to onset of action: 30-60 minutes

AEs: Rarely sedation at high doses

GRAS: Yes

Melatonin at a glance:
May address: Sleep parameters in the setting of ADHD; mitigates adverse effects of stimulant medication on sleep

Dose: 1-6mg at bedtime

Time to onset of action: 30-60 minutes

AEs: See full details

GRAS: No

Possible MOA: Possibly GABAergic

Magnesium at a glance:
May address: Sleep difficulties in a number of settings (not ADHD specifically)

Dose: 6-9mg per kilogram of body weight at bedtime

Time to onset of action: 30-60 minutes

AEs: Sedation and loose stools, also see full PDR entry

GRAS: Yes

Possible MOA: Neurotransmitter synthesis, GABAergic, serotonergic

Concurrent use of essential nutrients is implemented in a stepwise fashion with four to five days between adding each supplement. Start by addressing known deficiencies. See full prescribing considerations for each.

Omega-3 fats at a glance:
May address: Inattention, hyperactivity, oppositionality, aggression

Dose: 1000-5000mg EPA daily

Time to onset: 2-4 weeks

AEs: GI upset, fishy aftertaste (see full details)

GRAS: Yes

Prescription forms: Yes

Possible MOA: IIO axis, membrane-lipid therapy, dopaminergic, serotonergic

Omega-3 fats/EPA: Start with a target dose of approximately 1000 to 1500mg of EPA per day in the form of a high-potency softgel or liquid. Higher doses (5000mg or more) may be required for a clinical response. Allow two to four weeks for response time.

Brands of high-potency omega-3 softgels:
A. Thorne Super EPA Pro contains EPA 650mg and DHA 100mg per softgel

B. Vitamin Shoppe Omega-3 Fish Oil 735 EPA contains EPA 735mg and DHA 165mg per softgel

C. NutriGold triple strength fish oil contains EPA 750mg and DHA 250mg per softgel

Brands of high-potency omega-3 liquid:
A. Nordic Naturals Ultimate Omega XTRA contains EPA 2000mg and DHA 1000mg per *teaspoon* (when very high doses of 5-10g every day are attempted, this may be the best choice)

B. Barlean's Ultra High Potency Omega Swirl contains EPA 910mg and DHA 590mg per *tablespoon* (apparently does not taste fishy at all)

C. Vegan sourced DHA and EPA (produced from yeast) by Pure Encapsulations

Magnesium at a glance:
May address: Inattention, hyperactivity, aggression; anecdotal for sleep

Dose: 6-9mg per kilogram of body weight divided twice a day, with larger dose at bedtime

Time to onset of action: 30-60 minutes for sedative effects; 2-4 months for ADHD symptoms

AEs: Sedation and loose stools, see full PDR entry

GRAS: Yes

Possible MOA: Neurotransmitter and essential fatty acid synthesis, GABAergic, serotonergic

Magnesium and vitamin B6: Use Mg citrate, Mg glycinate, Mg taurate, or Mg threonate weight based at 6mg per kilogram of body weight per day along with vitamin B6 (preferably in the form of P5P) weight based at 0.6mg per kilogram of body weight per day. Higher doses of magnesium may be necessary for clinical response. Allow two to four months for response time. It can cause sedation, and evening dosing may be necessary.

Zinc at a glance:
May address: Optimize therapeutic effects of stimulants, decrease affective blunting associated with stimulants

Dose: Age based (see full details), twice daily dosing is preferable

Time to onset of action: Possibly 3-5 weeks

AEs: See PDR

GRAS: Yes

Prescription forms: Yes

Possible MOA: Neurotransmitter and essential fatty acid synthesis

Zinc: Ideally, zinc should be prescribed only if there is evidence of deficiency on laboratory test results. Zinc glycinate or gluconate has less GI upset than zinc sulfate does and may be more absorbable. For children four to eight years old, use 5 to 12mg per day, ideally divided twice a day (morning and early afternoon); for those nine to 13 years old, use 8 to 23mg per day; for those 14 to 18 years old, use 11 to 34mg per day; and for those 19 years old or older, use 11 to 40mg per day. Zinc may allow for a lower dose of stimulant medication and address the affective blunting associated with stimulants.

Iron at a glance:
May address: Inattention, hyperactivity, conduct problems, anxiety if levels of ferritin are low; may allow for lower dose of stimulant medication

Dose: Weight based and time limited if levels of ferritin are low (see full details)

AEs: Constipation with some formulations (see PDR)

GRAS: Yes

Prescription forms: Yes

Possible MOA: Neurotransmitter synthesis, dopamine transporter expression

Iron: Iron should be supplemented only in patients with low serum ferritin levels. Use ferrous sulfate, gluconate, or fumarate weight based in children 3 to 6mg per kilogram of body weight per day and 60mg per day in adolescents. Treat for one month, and then recheck levels. Continue treatment for two to three months after laboratory test result levels are corrected, and then recheck every six months. Iron may allow for a lower dose of stimulant medication.

Vitamin D3 at a glance:
May address: No direct evidence for efficacy in ADHD

Dose: Only supplemented if 25-hydroxyvitamin D is low (see full details)

AEs: See PDR

Vitamin D3: Vitamin D3 should be supplemented in patients who have low levels as indicated by laboratory test results. Serum levels should be greater than 20ng/ml, but 32ng/ml may be the true limit for sufficiency. When levels are very low, supplemental doses of up to 5000 units per day may be required. It is suggested that at supplemental doses greater than 400 units per day (the minimum daily requirement), 30 to 75mg of elemental calcium be prescribed daily (this translates to approximately 150-350mg of calcium citrate). One to two weeks after starting vitamin D therapy, this dose of calcium may be decreased by 50%. Vitamin D levels should be rechecked after three months and then annually.[831]

Probiotics at a glance:
May address: Indirect evidence of efficacy in addressing increased oxidative stress associated with ADHD, allergic rhinitis associated with ADHD, and food allergies associated with ADHD

Dose: At least 5-10 billion CFUs of broad-spectrum probiotics daily (see full details)

AEs: See full details

GRAS: Yes, some strains (and many more by European standards)

Prescription forms: Yes

Medical food: Yes

Possible MOA: IIO axis

Probiotics: Start with a broad-spectrum probiotic supplement that contains a variety of microorganisms dosed to provide at least 5 billion CFUs in children and 10 billion CFUs in adults given with or shortly after meals for a minimum of two to three weeks. Higher doses may be used for improved clinical response. Probiotics may also address symptoms of allergic rhinitis and food allergies.

Recommended Probiotic Products:
A. ProThera's Ther-Biotic Complete Capsules or Powder: This broad-spectrum product contains *B bifidum, B breve, B lactis, B longum, L acidophilus, L breve, L bulgaricus, L casei, L paracasei, L plantarum, L rhamnosus,* and *S thermophilus.*

B. Ultra Jarro-Dophilus: This broad-spectrum product contains 40 billion CFUs per capsule of *B breve, B lactis, B longum, L acidophilus, L casei, L lactis, L paracasei, L plantarum, L rhamnosus,* and *L salivarius.* It tends to be more widely available than ProThera products.

Multivitamins at a glance:
Multivitamins: Iron-free products with activated B vitamins and absorbable forms of zinc are preferred. Be careful not to exceed the acceptable upper daily intakes of fat-soluble vitamins (A, E, D, K) and minerals. Prescribing an adult multivitamin to children is acceptable provided the dose is adjusted for age or weight.

Recommended Multivitamin/Mineral Products:
A. VitaPrime by ProThera

B. Multi t/d by Pure Encapsulations

Essential nutrients are followed by serial use of metabolic nutrients, which may later be combined if they are only partially effective individually. See full prescribing considerations for each.

PS at a glance:

May address: Inattention, hyperactivity, impulsivity, oppositionality, mood dysregulation

Dose: 100-400mg in the morning, titrated gradually

Time to onset of action: 2-15 weeks

AEs: May increase dopamine and aggravate psychosis, see full details

GRAS: Yes

Medical food: Yes

Possible MOA: IIO axis, membrane-lipid therapy, cholinergic, dopaminergic, glutamate modulation

Phosphatidylserine: Start with 100mg every morning or 100mg twice a day (morning and early afternoon), then titrate slowly up to a total daily dose of 400mg, if necessary. Higher doses of up to 700mg every day may be used in some cases. Allow two to four weeks for response time. It may be activating, so use caution if the patient is also taking a stimulant and avoid dosing late in the day (and possibly even in the afternoon) if activation leads to insomnia. PS may increase dopamine and aggravate psychotic symptoms,[832] so be aware of any history of psychosis and/or mania in the patient or family and avoid in schizophrenia.

ALCAR at a glance:

May address: Inattention, hyperactivity; addresses irritability and headaches associated with stimulant medications

Dose: 500-3000mg in the morning

Time to onset of action: Approximately 6 weeks (possibly less)

AEs: Increased dopamine may exacerbate mania and psychosis, possible neuroendocrine and hormonal effects, see full details and PDR entry

GRAS: Yes

Prescription forms: Yes

Possible MOA: IIO axis, membrane-lipid therapy, cholinergic, dopaminergic, noradrenergic, serotonergic

Acetyl-L-carnitine (ALCAR): Start with 500mg every morning and titrate slowly up to 1500mg every morning or more (possibly up to 3000mg every morning). Allow two to four weeks' response time. Watch for activation and irritability. Use caution with stimulants. There is a case report of psychosis in a patient with bipolar disorder, possibly secondary to increased dopamine.[833] It may be wise to monitor levels of LH and prolactin, especially in pediatric patients.

NAC at a glance:

May address: Indirect evidence and inattention in SLE patients only

Dose: 150-2400mg twice daily (morning and early afternoon)

Time to onset of action: Unknown—days to 3 months

AEs: See PDR entry

GRAS: Yes

Prescription forms: Yes

Possible MOA: IIO axis, glutamate modulation

N-acetylcysteine: Start with 150mg twice daily (morning and early afternoon) in children and 300mg twice daily in adults.

Then titrate slowly to a maximum dose of 2400 twice daily. It may take several weeks for therapeutic effects to become apparent. Evidence for efficacy of NAC in treating ADHD is mainly extrapolated from its role as an antioxidant and glutamate modulator.

After metabolic nutrients, serial use of certain herbs in some populations cycled four to six weeks on and at least two weeks off may be appropriate. See full prescribing considerations for each.

Pycnogenol at a glance:
May address: Inattention

Dose: 1-2mg per kilogram of body weight in the morning or divided twice daily

Time to onset: May take up to 2 months

AEs: See full details

GRAS: Yes

Possible MOA: Antioxidant, membrane-lipid therapy

Pycnogenol: Start with 1mg per kilogram of body weight per day. This may be maintained for approximately one month. Efficacy may be increased by dividing doses twice a day (every morning and early afternoon) and increasing the dose to 2mg per kilogram of body weight per day or more. A full therapeutic effect may take up to two months or longer.

GB at a glance:
May address: Inattention, hyperactivity, anxiety

Dose: 80-200mg per day of standardized extract

Time to onset of action: 4-6 weeks

AEs: Possible endocrine or hormonal effects (see full details)

GRAS: No

Possible MOA: IIO axis, membrane-lipid therapy, cholinergic, dopaminergic, noradrenergic, GABAergic

Ginkgo biloba: Ginkgo biloba extract in the form of EGb 761 or other extract that is independently monitored for potency and purity may be used in adults with ADHD at doses ranging from 80 to 240mg per day divided into two or three doses daily. Because of concerns over hormonal effects, GB may be seen as conservatively contraindicated in children or may be used with caution at doses ranging from 80 to 120mg or more. Monitoring of serum testosterone levels and liver function may be advised in both children and adult populations. When given with stimulants and other dopaminergic medications or supplements, GB could have additive effects. Caution is advised.

White peony at a glance:
May address: No evidence of efficacy in treating ADHD as an individual agent

Dose: Unknown

Time to onset of action: Unknown

AEs: Possible hormonal effects (see full details)

GRAS: No

Possible MOA: IIO axis, cholinergic, noradrenergic

White peony: Starting with a low dose of liquid extract and titrating slowly would be a conservative approach. Its likely mechanisms of action suggest that it may be best to dose peony in the morning and possibly midday, but avoid dosing late in the day, as it may be activating. Its ability to increase norepinephrine could potentiate the effects of stimulant medications that may be prescribed. In vitro research indicates that it dependently decreases the production of testosterone in ovarian tissue. Therefore, it may be conservatively contraindicated or testosterone levels could be monitored.

Ashwagandha at a glance:
May address: No evidence of efficacy in treating ADHD as an individual agent

Dose: Unknown

Time to onset of action: Unknown

AEs: Possible neuroendocrine and hormonal effects (see full details)

GRAS: No

Possible MOA: IIO axis, cholinergic, dopaminergic, GABAergic, serotonergic

Ashwagandha: Because of its gonadotropic and possibly thyrotropic effects, it should either be avoided in children and adolescents or testosterone, LH, and thyroid levels should be monitored. Administration to adults may be appropriate, with doses ranging from 300 to 500mg per day of extract commonly standardized to 1.5% withanolides, 6 to 12ml per day of 1:2 fluid extract, or up to 3 to 6g per day of dried root. Evening dosing is recommended because it can be sedating.

Gotu kola at a glance:
May address: No evidence of efficacy in treating ADHD as an individual agent

Dose: Unknown

Time to onset of action: Unknown

AEs: Possible neuroendocrine and hormonal effects (see full details)

GRAS: No

Possible MOA: IIO axis, cholinergic, dopaminergic, noradrenergic, GABAergic, serotonergic

Gotu kola: Avoiding use in children is prudent. However, it may be used with caution in adults with ADHD. Common doses of extract range from 60 to 120mg per day.[834]

Spirulina at a glance:
May address: Inattention, hyperactivity, impulsivity (when considered as a form of multinutrient therapy), and allergic rhinitis

Dose: 250mg to several grams per day

Time to onset of action: Unknown, possibly weeks to months

AEs: GI upset (see full details)

GRAS: Yes (considered safe even for infants and young children)

Possible MOA when considered as a form of multinutrient therapy: IIO axis, neurotransmitter synthesis, membrane-lipid therapy

Spirulina: As a multinutrient approach to treating ADHD and to target comorbid symptoms of allergic rhinitis, spirulina may be given at doses ranging from 250mg to several grams per day.

Bacopa at a glance:
May address: Cognitive performance in the setting of ADHD in children

Dose: 100mg per day of extract

Time to onset of action: 12 weeks

AEs: Antifertility and antispermatogenic effects (see full details)

GRAS: No

Possible MOA: IIO axis, cholinergic, modulates glutamate, serotonergic

Bacopa: Antifertility concerns in males make it contraindicated in children until more safety data are available. In adults, doses range from 5 to 10g per day of raw herb powder to 200 to 400mg per day of extract standardized to 2% bacosides.[835]

Lemon balm at a glance:
May address: No evidence of efficacy in treating ADHD as an individual agent

Dose: Unknown

AEs: Possibly sedating, possible interaction with thyroid medications (see full details)

Time to onset of action: unknown

GRAS: Yes

Possible MOA: Antioxidant, cholinergic, GABAergic

Lemon balm: Commonly used doses of lemon balm extract in adults are 300 to 600mg per day and in children are 75 to 300mg per day.

Chamomile at a glance:
May address: Inattention, hyperactivity, impulsivity

May allow for lower dose of stimulant medication when used adjunctively

May protect against tics associated with stimulant medication

Dose: 100mg extract and 190mg of essential oil per day

Time to onset of action: 4 weeks

AEs: Sedation, allergic reactions, possible antithymus activity at high doses for long periods (see full details)

GRAS: Yes

Possible MOA: IIO axis, dopaminergic, noradrenergic, glutamate modulation, GABAergic

Chamomile: Because of potential cytotoxicity to thymus and
possibly other cells, chamomile should not be used at high
doses multiple times per day over long periods until safety
studies have been performed. When used periodically in the
form of tea or extract, it appears to be a safe and possibly effective treatment for occasional anxiety and insomnia.

Passionflower at a glance:
May address: No evidence of efficacy in treating ADHD as an
individual agent

Dose: Unknown

Time to onset of action: Unknown

AEs: Possible antithyroid activity, potential toxicity of some
constituents, sedation (see full details)

GRAS: Yes

Possible MOA: IIO axis, cholinergic, dopaminergic, noradrenergic, GABAergic, serotonergic

Passionflower: Because of concerns over passionflower's
narrow therapeutic index, antithyroid activity, possible toxicity
to human cells that express the enzyme myeloperoxidase, and
potential toxic effects of harmane, high-dose use for long durations is not recommended until further safety studies are available. Once deemed to be safe, vitexin may be the component of
PI that could be the most useful for ADHD symptoms. It is likely
safe for short-term use as an antianxiety/sedative/hypnotic
agent, as well as for the mental symptoms associated with
opiate withdrawal. It is often ingested as tea made from dried
leaves or as a liquid or powdered extract often standardized to
certain percentages of vitexin or isovitexin.

III. Follow-Up

1. If results are lacking, revisit dietary interventions, especially restriction diets.

2. Consider monitoring appropriate laboratory test results and correlate with clinical improvements.

3. Consider the use of prescription medications, including stimulants, atomoxetine, and/or alpha-2 agonists.

4. Adjust doses of supplements according to increases in body mass or age.

About the Author

Emanuel Frank, MD is a child and adult psychiatrist who has practiced in the San Francisco Bay Area since 2004. Dr. Frank integrates nutritional interventions with pharmacotherapy and takes a predominantly psychodynamic approach in psycho-therapy to help create significant and enduring change in client's lives. He is a board-certified psychiatrist who holds a masters degree in psychology from Pepperdine University, an MD from Ross University, and has completed residency in adult psychiatry at Harvard University and fellowship in child and adolescent psychiatry at Stanford University.

Notes

Chapter 2

1   Willcutt EG. The prevalence of DSM-IV attention-deficit/hyperactivity disorder: a meta-analytic review. *Neurotherapeutics.* 2012 Jul;9(3):490-9. doi: 10.1007/s13311-012-0135-8.

2   Bálint S, Czobor P, Mészáros A, Simon V, Bitter I. Neuropsychological impairments in adult attention deficit hyperactivity disorder: a literature review. *Psychiatr Hung.* 2008;23(5):324-35.

3   Rao TS, Asha MR, Ramesh BN, Rao KS. Understanding nutrition, depression and mental illnesses. *Indian J Psychiatry.* 2008 Apr;50(2):77-82. doi: 10.4103/0019-5545.42391.

4   Lakhan SE, Vieira KF. Nutritional therapies for mental disorders. *Nutr J.* 2008;7:2.

Chapter 4

5   What is a dietary supplement? U.S. Food and Drug Administration website. http://www.fda.gov/AboutFDA/Transparency/Basics/ucm195635.htm. Updated December 30, 2009.

6   Forsythe P, Sudo N, Dinan T, Taylor VH, Bienenstock J. Mood and gut feelings. *Brain Behav Immun.* 2010 Jan;24(1):9-16.

7   Schuchardt JP, Huss M, Stauss-Grabo M, Hahn A. Significance of long-chain polyunsaturated fatty acids (PUFAs) for the development and behaviour of children. *Eur J Pediatr.* 2010 Feb;169(2):149-64.

8   Facts About the Current Good Manufacturing Practices (CGMPs). U.S. Food and Drug Administration website.http://www.fda.gov/Drugs/DevelopmentApprovalProcess/Manufacturing/ucm169105.htm. Updated January 6, 2015.

9   About Us. GMP Certification Organization website. http://www.gmp-compliance.org/gmp-gdp-certification-programme.

10   Dietary Supplement Certification: Quality and Safety Provider. NSF International, The Public Health and Safety Organization website. http://www.nsf.org/services/by-industry/dietary-supplements.

11   Dietary Supplements. U.S. Food and Drug Administration website. http://www.fda.gov/Food/DietarySupplements/. Updated February 26, 2014.

12   Guidance for Industry: FDA's Implementation of "Qualified Health Claims": Questions and Answers; Final Guidance. U.S. Food and Drug Administration website. http://www.fda.gov/Food/GuidanceRegulation/GuidanceDocumentsRegulatoryInformation/ucm053843.htm. May 12, 2006.

Chapter 5

13   Bachman JL, Reedy J, Subar AF, Krebs-Smith S. Sources of food group intakes among the US population, 2001-2002. *J Am Diet Assoc.* 2008 May;108(5):804-14. doi: 10.1016/j.jada.2008.02.026.

14   O'Neil CE, Keast DR, Fulgoni VL, Nicklas TA. Food sources of energy and nutrients among adults in the US: NHANES 2003–2006. *Nutrients.* 2012 Dec 19;4(12):2097-120. doi: 10.3390/nu4122097.

15   O'Neil CE, Keast DR, Fulgoni VL, Nicklas TA. Food sources of energy and nutrients among adults in the US: NHANES 2003–2006. *Nutrients*. 2012 Dec 19;4(12):2097-120. doi: 10.3390/nu4122097.

16   Muñoz KA, Krebs-Smith SM, Ballard-Barbash R, Cleveland LE. Food intakes of US children and adolescents compared with recommendations. *Pediatrics*. 1997 Sep;100(3 Pt 1):323-9.

17   Hotz C, Gibson RS. Traditional food-processing and preparation practices to enhance the bioavailability of micronutrients in plant-based diets. *J Nutr*. 2007;137(4):1097-100.

18   Hotz C, Gibson RS. Traditional food-processing and preparation practices to enhance the bioavailability of micronutrients in plant-based diets. *J Nutr*. 2007;137(4):1097-100.

19   Rao TS, Asha MR, Ramesh BN, Rao KS. Understanding nutrition, depression and mental illnesses. *Indian J Psychiatry*. 2008 Apr;50(2):77-82. doi: 10.4103/0019-5545.42391.

20   Lakhan SE, Vieira KF. Nutritional therapies for mental disorders. *Nutr J*. 2008;7:2.

21   Rucklidge JJ, Johnstone J, Kaplan BJ. Nutrient supplementation approaches in the treatment of ADHD. *Expert Rev Neurother*. 2009 Apr;9(4):461-76. doi: 10.1586/ern.09.7.

22   Ames BN, Elson-Schwab I, Silver EA. High-dose vitamin therapy stimulates variant enzymes with decreased coenzyme binding affinity (increased K(m)): relevance to genetic disease and polymorphisms. *Am J Clin Nutr*. 2002 Apr;75(4):616-58.

23   Ames BN, Elson-Schwab I, Silver EA. High-dose vitamin therapy stimulates variant enzymes with decreased coenzyme binding affinity (increased K(m)): relevance to genetic disease and polymorphisms. *Am J Clin Nutr*. 2002 Apr;75(4):616-58.

24   Rucklidge JJ, Johnstone J, Kaplan BJ. Nutrient supplementation approaches in the treatment of ADHD. *Expert Rev Neurother*. 2009 Apr;9(4):461-76. doi: 10.1586/ern.09.7.

25   Ames BN, Elson-Schwab I, Silver EA. High-dose vitamin therapy stimulates variant enzymes with decreased coenzyme binding affinity (increased K(m)): relevance to genetic disease and polymorphisms. *Am J Clin Nutr*. 2002 Apr;75(4):616-58.

26   Tsaluchidu S, Cocchi M, Tonello L, Puri BK. Fatty acids and oxidative stress in psychiatric disorders. *BMC Psychiatry*. 2008 Apr 17;8 Suppl 1:S5.

27   Tsaluchidu S, Cocchi M, Tonello L, Puri BK. Fatty acids and oxidative stress in psychiatric disorders. *BMC Psychiatry*. 2008 Apr 17;8 Suppl 1:S5.

28   Christmas DM, Potokar J, Davies SJ. A biological pathway linking inflammation and depression: activation of indoleamine 2,3-dioxygenase. *Neuropsychiatr Dis Treat*. 2011;7:431-9.

29   Capuron L, Miller AH. Immune system to brain signaling: neuropsychopharmacological implications. *Pharmacol Ther*. 2011 May;130(2):226-38.

30   Membrane-lipid therapy. Universitat del les Illes Balears website. http://www.uib.cat/depart/dba/cellbiology/lipid.html. Accessed 2009.

31   Wong-Ekkabut J, Xu Z, Triampo W, Tang IM, Tieleman DP, Monticelli L. Effect of lip-

id peroxidation on the properties of lipid bilayers: a molecular dynamics study. *Biophys J.* 2007 Dec 15;93(12):4225-36.

32   Rojas P, Serrano-García N, Medina-Campos ON, Pedraza-Chaverri J, Ogren SO, Rojas C. Antidepressant-like effect of a Ginkgo biloba extract (EGb761) in the mouse forced swimming test: role of oxidative stress. *Neurochem Int.* 2011 Oct;59(5):628-36. doi: 10.1016/j.neuint.2011.05.007.

33   Leistner E, Drewke C. Ginkgo biloba and ginkgotoxin. *J Nat Prod.* 2010 Jan;73(1):86-92. doi: 10.1021/np9005019.

34   Gałecki P, Szemraj J, Bieńkiewicz M, Florkowski A, Gałecka E. Lipid peroxidation and antioxidant protection in patients during acute depressive episodes and in remission after fluoxetine treatment. *Pharmacol Rep.* 2009 May-Jun;61(3):436-47.

35   Versace A, Andreazza AC, Young LT, et al. Elevated serum measures of lipid peroxidation and abnormal prefrontal white matter in euthymic bipolar adults: toward peripheral biomarkers of bipolar disorder. *Mol Psychiatry.* 2013 Jan 29. doi: 10.1038/mp.2012.188.

36   Versace A, Andreazza AC, Young LT, et al. Elevated serum measures of lipid peroxidation and abnormal prefrontal white matter in euthymic bipolar adults: toward peripheral biomarkers of bipolar disorder. *Mol Psychiatry.* 2013 Jan 29. doi: 10.1038/mp.2012.188.

37   Bulut M, Selek S, Bez Y, et al. Reduced PON1 enzymatic activity and increased lipid hydroperoxide levels that point out oxidative stress in generalized anxiety disorder. *J Affect Disord.* 2013 Sep 25;150(3):829-33. doi: 10.1016/j.jad.2013.03.011.

38   Huang MC, Chen CH, Peng FC, Tang SH, Chen CC. Alterations in oxidative stress status during early alcohol withdrawal in alcoholic patients. *J Formos Med Assoc.* 2009 Jul;108(7):560-9. doi: 10.1016/S0929-6646(09)60374-0.

39   Gulec M, Ozkol H, Selvi Y, et al. Oxidative stress in patients with primary insomnia. *Prog Neuropsychopharmacol Biol Psychiatry.* 2012 Jun 1;37(2):247-51. doi: 10.1016/j.pnpbp.2012.02.011.

40   Bulut M, Selek S, Bez Y, et al. Lipid peroxidation markers in adult attention deficit hyperactivity disorder: new findings for oxidative stress. *Psychiatry Res.* 2013;209(3):638-42.

41   PV Escribá. Membrane-lipid therapy: a new approach in molecular medicine. *Trends Mol Med.* 2006 Jan;12(1):34-43.

Chapter 6

42   Lakhan SE, Vieira KF. Nutritional therapies for mental disorders. *Nutr J.* 2008 Jan 21;7:2. doi: 10.1186/1475-2891-7-2.

43   Lakhan SE, Vieira KF. Nutritional therapies for mental disorders. *Nutr J.* 2008 Jan 21;7:2. doi: 10.1186/1475-2891-7-2.

44   Medical Foods Guidance Documents & Regulatory Information. U.S. Food and Drug Administration website. http://www.fda.gov/food/guidanceregulation/guidancedocumentsregulatoryinformation/medicalfoods/default.htm. Updated August 21, 2013.

45   Lakhan SE, Vieira KF. Nutritional therapies for mental disorders. *Nutr J.* 2008 Jan 21;7:2. doi: 10.1186/1475-2891-7-2.

Chapter 7

46   Thapar A, Cooper M, Eyre O, Langley K. Practitioner Review: What have we learnt about the causes of ADHD? *J Child Psychol Psychiatry.* 2013 Jan;54(1):3-16. doi: 10.1111/j.1469-7610.2012.02611.x.

47   Konrad K, Eickhoff SB. Is the ADHD brain wired differently? A review on structural and functional connectivity in attention deficit hyperactivity disorder. *Hum Brain Mapp.* 2010 Jun;31(6):904-16. doi: 10.1002/hbm.21058.

48   Thapar A, Cooper M, Eyre O, Langley K. Practitioner Review: What have we learnt about the causes of ADHD? *J Child Psychol Psychiatry.* 2013 Jan;54(1):3-16. doi: 10.1111/j.1469-7610.2012.02611.x.

49   Konrad K, Eickhoff SB. Is the ADHD brain wired differently? A review on structural and functional connectivity in attention deficit hyperactivity disorder. *Hum Brain Mapp.* 2010 Jun;31(6):904-16. doi: 10.1002/hbm.21058.

50   Thapar A, Cooper M, Eyre O, Langley K. Practitioner Review: What have we learnt about the causes of ADHD? *J Child Psychol Psychiatry.* 2013 Jan;54(1):3-16. doi: 10.1111/j.1469-7610.2012.02611.x.

51   Waschbusch DA, Pelham WE Jr, Waxmonsky J, Johnston C. Are there placebo effects in the medication treatment of children with attention-deficit hyperactivity disorder? *J Dev Behav Pediatr.* 2009;30(2):158-68.

52   Wilens TE, Spencer TJ, Biederman J. A review of the pharmacotherapy of adults with attention-deficit/hyperactivity disorder. *J Atten Disord.* 2002;5(4):189-202.

53   Chovanová Z, Muchová J, Sivonová M, et al. Effect of polyphenolic extract, Pycnogenol, on the level of 8-oxoguanine in children suffering from attention deficit/ hyperactivity disorder. *Free Radic Res.* 2006 Sep;40(9):1003-10.

54   Joseph N, Zhang-James Y, Perl A, Faraone SV. Oxidative stress and ADHD: a meta-analysis. *J Atten Disord.* 2015;19(11):915-24.

55   Bulut M, Selek S, Gergerlioglu HS, et al. Malondialdehyde levels in adult attention-deficit hyperactivity disorder. *J Psychiatry Neurosci.* 2007 Nov;32(6):435-8.

56   Selek S, Bulut M, Ocak AR, Kalenderoğlu A, Savaş HA. Evaluation of total oxidative status in adult attention deficit hyperactivity disorder and its diagnostic implications. *J Psychiatr Res.* 2012 Apr;46(4):451-5.

57   Oztop D, Altun H, Baskol G, Ozsoy S. Oxidative stress in children with attention deficit hyperactivity disorder. *Clin Biochem.* 2012;45(10-11):745-8.

58   Spahis S, Vanasse M, Bélanger SA, Ghadirian P, Grenier E, Levy E. Lipid profile, fatty acid composition and pro- and anti-oxidant status in pediatric patients with attention-deficit/hyperactivity disorder. *Prostaglandins Leukot Essent Fatty Acids.* 2008;79(1-2):47-53.

59   Essawy H, El-Ghohary I, El-Missiry A, Kahla O, Soliman A, El-Rashidi O. Oxidative stress in attention deficit hyperactivity disorder patients. *Curr Psychiatr.* 2009;16(1):56-69.

60   Dvoráková M, Jezová D, Blazícek P, et al. Urinary catecholamines in children with attention deficit hyperactivity disorder (ADHD): modulation by a polyphenolic extract from pine bark (pycnogenol). *Nutr Neurosci.* 2007 Jun-Aug;10(3-4):151-7.

Notes

61   Trebatická J, Kopasová S, Hradecná Z, et al. Treatment of ADHD with French maritime pine bark extract, Pycnogenol. *Eur Child Adolesc Psychiatry.* 2006 Sep;15(6):329-35.

62   Martins MR, Reinke A, Petronilho FC, Gomes KM, Dal-Pizzol F, Quevedo J. Methylphenidate treatment induces oxidative stress in young rat brain. *Brain Res.* 2006 Mar 17;1078(1):189-97.

63   Silva AP, Martins T, Baptista S, Gonçalves J, Agasse F, Malva JO. Brain injury associated with widely abused amphetamines: neuroinflammation, neurogenesis and blood-brain barrier. *Curr Drug Abuse Rev.* 2010 Dec 1;3(4):239-54.

64   Govitrapong P, Boontem P, Kooncumchoo P, et al. Increased blood oxidative stress in amphetamine users. *Addict Biol.* 2010 Jan;15(1):100-2.

65   El-Tawil OS, Abou-Hadeed AH, El-Bab MF, Shalaby AA. d-Amphetamine-induced cytotoxicity and oxidative stress in isolated rat hepatocytes. *Pathophysiology.* 2011 Sep;18(4):279-85.

66   Sae-Ung K, Uéda K, Govitrapong P, Phansuwan-Pujito P. Melatonin reduces the expression of alpha-synuclein in the dopamine containing neuronal regions of amphetamine-treated postnatal rats. *J Pineal Res.* 2012 Jan;52(1):128-37. doi: 10.1111/j.1600-079X.2011.00927.x.

67   Valvassori SS, Petronilho FC, Réus GZ, et al. Effect of N-acetylcysteine and/or deferoxamine on oxidative stress and hyperactivity in an animal model of mania. *Prog Neuropsychopharmacol Biol Psychiatry.* 2008;32(4):1064-8.

68   Schmidt AJ, Krieg JC, Clement HW, Gebhardt S, Schulz E, Heiser P. Impact of drugs approved for treating ADHD on the cell survival and energy metabolism: an in-vitro study in human neuronal and immune cells. *J Psychopharmacol.* 2010 Dec;24(12):1829-33.

69   Settipane RA. Complications of allergic rhinitis. *Allergy Asthma Proc.* 1999 Jul-Aug;20(4):209-13.

70   Castellanos FX, Lee PP, Sharp W, et al. Developmental trajectories of brain volume abnormalities in children and adolescents with attention-deficit/hyperactivity disorder. *JAMA.* 2002 Oct 9;288(14):1740-8.

71   Dvoráková M, Sivonová M, Trebatická J, et al. The effect of polyphenolic extract from pine bark, Pycnogenol on the level of glutathione in children suffering from attention deficit hyperactivity disorder (ADHD). *Redox Rep.* 2006;11(4):163-72.

72   Brawley A, Silverman B, Kearney S, et al. Allergic rhinitis in children with attention-deficit/hyperactivity disorder. *Ann Allergy Asthma Immunol.* 2004 Jun;92(6):663-7.

73   Settipane RA. Complications of allergic rhinitis. *Allergy Asthma Proc.* 1999 Jul-Aug;20(4):209-13.

74   Zamora J, Velásquez A, Troncoso L, Barra P, Guajardo K, Castillo Duran C. Zinc in the therapy of the attention-deficit/hyperactivity disorder in children. A preliminary randomized controlled trial. *Arch Latinoam Nutr.* 2011 Sep;61(3):242-6.

75   Chervin RD, Dillon JE, Bassetti C, Ganoczy DA, Pituch KJ. Symptoms of sleep disorders, inattention, and hyperactivity in children. *SLEEP.* 1997 Dec;20(12):1185-92.

76   Chervin RD, Dillon JE, Bassetti C, Ganoczy DA, Pituch KJ. Symptoms of sleep disorders, inattention, and hyperactivity in children. *SLEEP.* 1997 Dec;20(12):1185-92.

77   Chervin RD, Dillon JE, Bassetti C, Ganoczy DA, Pituch KJ. Symptoms of sleep disorders, inattention, and hyperactivity in children. *SLEEP.* 1997 Dec;20(12):1185-92.

78   Zamora J, Velásquez A, Troncoso L, Barra P, Guajardo K, Castillo-Duran C. Zinc in the therapy of the attention-deficit/hyperactivity disorder in children. A preliminary randomized controlled trial. *Arch Latinoam Nutr.* 2011 Sep;61(3):242-6.

79   Pesticides in the Diets of Infants and Children. US National Research Council, Committee on Pesticides in the Diets of Infants and Children. Washington, DC: National Academy Press; 1993.

80   Nigg JT, Lewis K, Edinger T, Falk M. Meta-analysis of attention-deficit/hyperactivity disorder or attention-deficit/hyperactivity disorder symptoms, restriction diet, and synthetic food color additives. *J Am Acad Child Adolesc Psychiatry.* 2012 Jan;51(1):86-97. e8.

81   Pelsser LM, Buitelaar JK, Savelkoul HF. ADHD as a (non) allergic hypersensitivity disorder: a hypothesis. *Pediatr Allergy Immunol.* 2009;20(2):107-12.

82   Kanny G. Atopic dermatitis in children and food allergy: combination or causality? Should avoidance diets be initiated? *Ann Dermatol Venereol.* 2005 Jan;132 Spec No 1:1S90-103.

83   Noorbala AA, Akhondzadeh S. Attention-deficit/hyperactivity disorder: etiology and pharmacotherapy. *Arch Iran Med.* 2006 Oct;9(4):374-80.

Chapter 8

84   Sharma A, Couture J. A review of the pathophysiology, etiology, and treatment of attention-deficit hyperactivity disorder (ADHD). *Ann Pharmacother.* 2014;48(2):209-25.

85   Arnsten AF. Stimulants: Therapeutic actions in ADHD. *Neuropsychopharmacology.* 2006 Nov;31(11):2376-83.

86   Newcorn JH, Kratochvil CJ, Allen AJ, et al. Atomoxetine and osmotically released methylphenidate for the treatment of attention deficit hyperactivity disorder: acute comparison and differential response. *Am J Psychiatry.* 2008 Jun;165(6):721-30. doi: 10.1176/appi.ajp.2007.05091676.

87   Noorbala AA, Akhondzadeh S. Attention-deficit/hyperactivity disorder: etiology and pharmacotherapy. *Arch Iran Med.* 2006 Oct;9(4):374-80.

88   Banerjee E, Nandagopal K. Does serotonin deficit mediate susceptibility to ADHD? *Neurochem Int.* 2015;82:52-68.

89   Ferguson HB, Pappas BA, Trites RL, Peters DA, Taub H. Plasma free and total tryptophan, blood serotonin, and the hyperactivity syndrome: no evidence for the serotonin deficiency hypothesis. *Biol Psychiatry.* 1981;16(3):231-8.

90   Dolina S, Margalit D, Malitsky S, Rabinkov A. Attention-deficit hyperactivity disorder (ADHD) as a pyridoxine-dependent condition: urinary diagnostic biomarkers. *Med Hypotheses.* 2014;82(1):111-6.

91   Patrick RP, Ames BN. Vitamin D and the omega-3 fatty acids control serotonin synthesis and action, part 2: relevance for ADHD, bipolar disorder, schizophrenia, and impulsive behavior. *FASEB J.* 2015;29(6):2207-2222.

92   Johansson J, Landgren M, Fernell E, et al. Altered tryptophan and alanine transport in fibroblasts from boys with attention-deficit/hyperactivity disorder (ADHD): an in vitro study. *Behav Brain Funct.* 2011;7:40.

Notes

93   Hoshino Y, Ohno Y, Yamamoto T, Kaneko M, Kumashiro H. Plasma free tryptophan concentration in children with attention deficit disorder. *Folia Psychiatr Neurol Jpn.* 1985;39(4):531-5.

94   Spivak B, Vered Y, Yoran-Hegesh R, et al. Circulatory levels of catecholamines, serotonin and lipids in attention deficit hyperactivity disorder. *Acta Psychiatr Scand.* 1999;99(4):300-4.

95   Bhagavan HN, Coleman M, Coursin DB. The effect of pyridoxine hydrochloride on blood serotonin and pyridoxal phosphate contents in hyperactive children. *Pediatrics.* 1975;55(3):437-41.

96   Gizer IR, Ficks C, Waldman ID. Candidate gene studies of ADHD: a meta-analytic review. *Hum Genet.* 2009;126(1):51-90.

97   Banerjee E, Nandagopal K. Does serotonin deficit mediate susceptibility to ADHD? *Neurochem Int.* 2015;82:52-68.

98   Gizer IR, Ficks C, Waldman ID. Candidate gene studies of ADHD: a meta-analytic review. *Hum Genet.* 2009;126(1):51-90.

99   Li J, Wang YF, Zhou RL, Yang L, Zhang HB, Wang B. Association between tryptophan hydroxylase gene polymorphisms and attention deficit hyperactivity disorder with or without learning disorder [in Chinese]. *Zhonghua Yi Xue Za Zhi.* 2003;83(24):2114-8.

100   Halmøy A, Johansson S, Winge I, McKinney JA, Knappskog PM, Haavik J. Attention-deficit/hyperactivity disorder symptoms in offspring of mothers with impaired serotonin production. *Arch Gen Psychiatry.* 2010;67(10):1033-43.

101   Sheehan K, Lowe N, Kirley A, et al. Tryptophan hydroxylase 2 (TPH2) gene variants associated with ADHD. *Mol Psychiatry.* 2005;10(10):944-9.

102   Gizer IR, Ficks C, Waldman ID. Candidate gene studies of ADHD: a meta-analytic review. *Hum Genet.* 2009;126(1):51-90.

103   Barrickman L, Noyes R, Kuperman S, Schumacher E, Verda M. Treatment of ADHD with fluoxetine: a preliminary trial. *J Am Acad Child Adolesc Psychiatry.* 1991;30(5):762-7.

104   Quintana H, Butterbaugh GJ, Purnell W, Layman AK. Fluoxetine monotherapy in attention-deficit/hyperactivity disorder and comorbid non-bipolar mood disorders in children and adolescents. *Child Psychiatry Hum Dev.* 2007;37(3):241-53.

105   Banerjee E, Nandagopal K. Does serotonin deficit mediate susceptibility to ADHD? *Neurochem Int.* 2015;82:52-68.

106   English BA, Hahn MK, Gizer IR, et al. Choline transporter gene variation is associated with attention-deficit hyperactivity disorder. *J Neurodev Disord.* 2009 Dec;1(4):252-63. doi: 10.1007/s11689-009-9033-8.

107   Ohmura Y, Tsutsui-Kimura I, Yoshioka M. Impulsive behavior and nicotinic acetylcholine receptors. *J Pharmacol Sci.* 2012;118(4):413-22.

108   Johansson J, Landgren M, Fernell E, Lewander T, Venizelos N. Decreased binding capacity (B (max)) of muscarinic acetylcholine receptors in fibroblasts from boys with attention-deficit/hyperactivity disorder (ADHD). *Atten Defic Hyperact Disord.* February 7, 2013.

109   English BA, Hahn MK, Gizer IR, et al. Choline transporter gene variation is associated with attention-deficit hyperactivity disorder. *J Neurodev Disord.* 2009 Dec;1(4):252-63. doi: 10.1007/s11689-009-9033-8.

110   Lee J, Laurin N, Crosbie J, et al. Association study of the nicotinic acetylcholine receptor alpha4 subunit gene, CHRNA4, in attention-deficit hyperactivity disorder. *Genes Brain Behav.* 2008 Feb;7(1):53-60.

111   English BA, Hahn MK, Gizer IR, et al. Choline transporter gene variation is associated with attention-deficit hyperactivity disorder. *J Neurodev Disord.* 2009 Dec;1(4):252-63. doi: 10.1007/s11689-009-9033-8.

112   Wilens TE, Decker MW. Neuronal nicotinic receptor agonists for the treatment of attention-deficit/hyperactivity disorder: focus on cognition. *Biochem Pharmacol.* 2007 Oct 15;74(8):1212-23.

113   Wilens TE, Biederman J, Wong J, Spencer TJ, Prince JB. Adjunctive donepezil in attention deficit hyperactivity disorder youth: case series. *J Child Adolesc Psychopharmacol.* 2000 Fall;10(3):217-22.

114   Doyle RL, Frazier J, Spencer TJ, Geller D, Biederman J, Wilens T. Donepezil in the treatment of ADHD-like symptoms in youths with pervasive developmental disorder: a case series. *J Atten Disord.* 2006 Feb;9(3):543-9.

115   Biederman J, Mick E, Faraone S, et al. A double-blind comparison of galantamine hydrogen bromide and placebo in adults with attention-deficit/hyperactivity disorder: a pilot study. *J Clin Psychopharmacol.* 2006 Apr;26(2):163-6.

116   Park S, Jung SW, Kim BN, et al. Association between the GRM7 rs3792452 polymorphism and attention deficit hyperactivity disorder in a Korean sample. *Behav Brain Funct.* 2013 Jan 7;9(1):1.

117   Rout UK, Mungan NK, Dhossche DM. Presence of GAD65 autoantibodies in the serum of children with autism or ADHD. *Eur Child Adolesc Psychiatry.* 2012 Mar;21(3):141-7. doi: 10.1007/s00787-012-0245-1.

118   Pozzi L, Baviera M, Sacchetti G, et al. Attention deficit induced by blockade of N-methyl D-aspartate receptors in the prefrontal cortex is associated with enhanced glutamate release and cAMP response element binding protein phosphorylation: role of metabotropic glutamate receptors 2/3. *Neuroscience.* 2011 Mar 10;176:336-48. doi: 10.1016/j.neuroscience.2010.11.060.

119   Hammerness P, Biederman J, Petty C, Henin A, Moore CM. Brain biochemical effects of methylphenidate treatment using proton magnetic spectroscopy in youth with attention-deficit hyperactivity disorder: a controlled pilot study. *CNS Neurosci Ther.* 2012 Jan;18(1):34-40. doi: 10.1111/j.1755-5949.2010.00226.x.

120   Hoerst M, Weber-Fahr W, Tunc-Skarka N, et al. Correlation of glutamate levels in the anterior cingulate cortex with self-reported impulsivity in patients with borderline personality disorder and healthy controls. *Arch Gen Psychiatry.* 2010 Sep;67(9):946-54. doi: 10.1001/archgenpsychiatry.2010.93.

121   Perlov E, Philipsen A, Matthies S, et al. Spectroscopic findings in attention-deficit/hyperactivity disorder: review and meta-analysis. *World J Biol Psychiatry.* 2009;10(4 Pt 2):355-65. doi: 10.1080/15622970802176032.

122   Ludolph AG, Udvardi PT, Schaz U, et al. Atomoxetine acts as an NMDA receptor

blocker in clinically relevant concentrations. *Br J Pharmacol.* 2010 May;160(2):283-91. doi: 10.1111/j.1476-5381.2010.00707.x.

123   Findling RL, McNamara NK, Stansbrey RJ, et al. A pilot evaluation of the safety, tolerability, pharmacokinetics, and effectiveness of memantine in pediatric patients with attention-deficit/hyperactivity disorder combined type. *J Child Adolesc Psychopharmacol.* 2007 Feb;17(1):19-33.

124   Adler LA, Kroon RA, Stein M, et al. A translational approach to evaluate the efficacy and safety of the novel AMPA receptor positive allosteric modulator org 26576 in adult attention-deficit/hyperactivity disorder. *Biol Psychiatry.* 2012 Dec 1;72(11):971-7. doi: 10.1016/j.biopsych.2012.05.012.

125   Jupp B, Caprioli D, Saigal N, et al. Dopaminergic and GABA-ergic markers of impulsivity in rats: evidence for anatomical localisation in ventral striatum and prefrontal cortex. *Eur J Neurosci.* 2013 Feb 1. doi: 10.1111/ejn.12146.

126   Edden RA, Crocetti D, Zhu H, Gilbert DL, Mostofsky SH. Reduced GABA concentration in attention-deficit/hyperactivity disorder. *Arch Gen Psychiatry.* 2012 Jul;69(7):750-3. doi: 10.1001/archgenpsychiatry.2011.2280.

127   Boy F, Evans CJ, Edden RA, et al. Dorsolateral prefrontal γ-aminobutyric acid in men predicts individual differences in rash impulsivity. *Biol Psychiatry.* 2011 Nov 1;70(9):866-72. doi: 10.1016/j.biopsych.2011.05.030.

128   Ludolph AG, Udvardi PT, Schaz U, et al. Atomoxetine acts as an NMDA receptor blocker in clinically relevant concentrations. *Br J Pharmacol.* 2010;160(2):283-91.

Chapter 9

129   Pliszka S; AACAP Work Group on Quality Issues. Practice parameter for the assessment and treatment of children and adolescents with attention-deficit/hyperactivity disorder. *J Am Acad Child Adolesc Psychiatry.* 2007;46(7):894-921.

130   Attention-deficit/hyperactivity disorder (ADHD). Centers for Disease Control and Prevention. http://www.cdc.gov/ncbddd/adhd/diagnosis.html. Accessed July 28, 2015.

131   Pliszka S; AACAP Work Group on Quality Issues. Practice parameter for the assessment and treatment of children and adolescents with attention-deficit/hyperactivity disorder. *J Am Acad Child Adolesc Psychiatry.* 2007;46(7):894-921.

132   Lyon MR, Kapoor MP, Juneja LR. The Effects of L-Theanine (Suntheanine®) on Objective Sleep Quality in Boys with Attention Deficit Hyperactivity Disorder (ADHD): a Randomized, Double-blind, Placebo-controlled Clinical Trial. *Altern Med Rev.* 2011 Dec;16(4):348-54.

133   Gruber R, Sadeh A, Raviv A. Instability of sleep patterns in children with attention-deficit/hyperactivity disorder. *J Am Acad Child Adolesc Psychiatry.* 2000 Apr;39(4):495-501.

134   Stein MA. Unravelling sleep problems in treated and untreated children with ADHD. *J Child Adolesc Psychopharmacol.* 1999;9(3):157-68.

Chapter 10

135   Kapoor R, Huang YS. Gamma linolenic acid: an antiinflammatory omega-6 fatty acid. *Curr Pharm Biotechnol.* 2006;7(6):531-4.

136   Simopoulos AP. Evolutionary aspects of diet: the omega-6/omega-3 ratio and the brain. *Mol Neurobiol.* 2011 Oct;44(2):203-15. doi: 10.1007/s12035-010-8162-0.

137   Simopoulos AP. The importance of the ratio of omega-6/omega-3 essential fatty acids. *Biomed Pharmacother*. 2002;56(8):365-79.

138   Protecting and Promoting *Your* Health: *Trans* Fat. U.S. Food and Drug Administration website. http://www.fda.gov/Food/ucm292278.htm. June 16, 2015.

139   Golomb BA, Evans MA, White HL, Dimsdale JE. Trans fat consumption and aggression. PLoS One. 2012;7(3):e32175. doi: 10.1371/journal.pone.0032175.

140   McAfee AJ, McSorley EM, Cuskelly GJ, et al. Red meat from animals offered a grass diet increases plasma and platelet n-3 PUFA in healthy consumers. *Br J Nutr*. 2011 Jan;105(1):80-9.

141   Głogowski R, Czauderna M, Rozbicka A, Krajewska KA, Clauss M. Fatty acid profile of hind leg muscle in female and male nutria (Myocastor coypus Mol.), fed green forage diet. *Meat Sci*. 2010 Jul;85(3):577-9.

142   Głogowski R, Czauderna M, Rozbicka A, Krajew- ska KA, Clauss M. Fatty acid profile of hind leg muscle in female and male nutria (Myocastor coypus Mol.), fed green forage diet. *Meat Sci*. 2010 Jul;85(3):577-9.

143   McAfee AJ, McSorley EM, Cuskelly GJ, et al. Red meat from animals offered a grass diet increases plasma and platelet n-3 PUFA in healthy consumers. *Br J Nutr*. 2011 Jan;105(1):80-9.

144   Hauswirth CB, Scheeder MR, Beer JH. High omega-3 fatty acid content in alpine cheese: the basis for an alpine paradox. *Circulation*. 2004 Jan 6;109(1):103-7.

145   Shields PG, Xu GX, Blot WJ, et al. Mutagens from heated Chinese and U.S. cooking oils. *J Natl Cancer Inst*. 1995;87(11):836-41.

146   Enig MG. Trans Fatty Acids Are Not Formed by Heating Vegetable Oils. Weston A. Price Foundation® website. http://www.westonaprice.org/know-your-fats/trans-fatty-acids-are-not-formed-by-heating-vegetable-oils. Updated February 24, 2004.

147   Langseth L, Dowd J. Glucose tolerance and hyperkinesis. *Food Cosmet Toxicol*. 1978 Apr;16(2):129-33.

148   Millichap JG, Yee MM. The diet factor in attention-deficit/hyperactivity disorder. *Pediatrics*. 2012 Feb;129(2):330-7. doi: 10.1542/peds.2011-2199.

149   Langseth L, Dowd J. Glucose tolerance and hyperkinesis. *Food Cosmet Toxicol*. 1978 Apr;16(2):129-33.

150   Furlong CE, Holland N, Richter RJ, Bradman A, Ho A, Eskenazi B. PON1 status of farmworker mothers and children as a predictor of organophosphate sensitivity. *Pharmacogenet Genomics*. 2006;16(3):183-90.

151   Weiss B. Vulnerability of children and the developing brain to neurotoxic hazards. *Environ Health Perspect*. 2000;108(suppl 3):375–381.

152   Barr DB, Bravo R, Weerasekera G, et al. Concentrations of dialkyl phosphate metabolites of organophosphorus pesticides in the US population. *Environ Health Perspect*. 2004;112(2):186–200.

153   Furlong CE, Holland N, Richter RJ, Bradman A, Ho A, Eskenazi B. PON1 status of farmworker mothers and children as a predictor of organophosphate sensitivity. *Pharmacogenet Genomics*. 2006;16(3):183–190.

154   Rauh VA, Garfinkel R, Perera FP, et al. Impact of prenatal chlorpyrifos exposure

on neurodevelopment in the first 3 years of life among inner-city children. *Pediatrics*.2006;118(6):e1845-59.

155   Grandjean P, Harari R, Barr DB, Debes F. Pesticide exposure and stunting as independent predictors of neurobehavioral deficits in Ecuadorian school children. *Pediatrics*. 2006;117(3):e546-56.

156   Xu X, Nembhard WN, Kan H, Kearney G, Zhang ZJ, Talbott EO. Urinary trichlorophenol levels and increased risk of attention deficit hyperactivity disorder among US school-aged children. *Occup Environ Med*. 2011 Aug;68(8):557-61.

157   Noorbala AA, Akhondzadeh S. Attention-deficit/hyperactivity disorder: etiology and pharmacotherapy. *Arch Iran Med*. 2006 Oct;9(4):374-80.

158   Pelsser LM, Buitelaar JK, Savelkoul HF. ADHD as a (non) allergic hypersensitivity disorder: a hypothesis. *Pediatr Allergy Immunol*. 2009;20(2):107-12.

159   Stevens LJ, Kuczek T, Burgess JR, Hurt E, Arnold LE. Dietary sensitivities and ADHD symptoms: thirty-five years of research. *Clin Pediatr (Phila)*. 2011 Apr;50(4):279-93.

160   Pelsser LM, Frankena K, Toorman J, Savelkoul HF, Dubois AE, Pereira RR, Haagen TA, Rommelse NN, Buitelaar JK. Effects of a restricted elimination diet on the behaviour of children with attention-deficit hyperactivity disorder (INCA study): a randomised controlled trial. *Lancet*. 2011 Feb 5;377(9764):494-503.

161   Nigg JT, Lewis K, Edinger T, Falk M. Meta-analysis of attention-deficit/hyperactivity disorder or attention-deficit/hyperactivity disorder symptoms, restriction diet, and synthetic food color additives. *J Am Acad Child Adolesc Psychiatry*. 2012 Jan;51(1):86-97.e8.

162   Furlong CE, Holland N, Richter RJ, Bradman A, Ho A, Eskenazi B. PON1 status of farmworker mothers and children as a predictor of organophosphate sensitivity. *Pharmacogenet Genomics*. 2006;16(3):183–190.

163   Marks AR, Harley K, Bradman A, et al. Organophosphate pesticide exposure and attention in young Mexican-American children: the CHAMACOS study. *Environ Health Perspect*. 2010;118(12):1768-74.

164   Bouchard MF, Bellinger DC, Wright RO, Weisskopf MG. Attention-deficit/hyperactivity disorder and urinary metabolites of organophosphate pesticides. *Pediatrics*. 2010;125(6):e1270-7.

165   Schantz SL, Widholm JJ, Rice DC. Effects of PCB exposure on neuropsychological function in children. *Environ Health Perspect*. 2003;111(3):357-576.

166   Sagiv SK, Thurston SW, Bellinger DC, Tolbert PE, Altshul LM, Korrick SA. Prenatal organochlorine exposure and behaviors associated with attention deficit hyperactivity disorder in school-aged children. *Am J Epidemiol*. 2010;171(5):593-601.

167   Schab DW, Trinh NH. Do artificial food colors promote hyperactivity in children with hyperactive syndromes? A meta-analysis of double-blind placebo-controlled trials. *J Dev Behav Pediatr*. 2004 Dec;25(6):423-34.

168   L-theanine. Monograph. *Altern Med Rev*. 2005 Jun;10(2):136-8.

169   US Food and Drug Administration website. http://www.fda.gov/ucm/groups/fdagov-public/@fdagov-foods-gen/documents/document/ucm263912.pdf. Accessed 2016.

170   US Food and Drug Administration website. http://www.fda.gov/ucm/groups/fda-gov-public/@fdagov-foods-gen/documents/document/ucm263912.pdf. Accessed 2016.

171   US Food and Drug Administration website. http://www.fda.gov/ucm/groups/fda-gov-public/@fdagov-foods-gen/documents/document/ucm263912.pdf. Accessed 2016.

172   Lyon MR, Kapoor MP, Juneja LR. The effects of L-theanine (Suntheanine®) on objective sleep quality in boys with attention deficit hyperactivity disorder (ADHD): a randomized, double-blind, placebo-controlled clinical trial. *Altern Med Rev.* 2011 Dec;16(4):348-54.

173   Bannai M, Kawai N, Nagao K, Nakano S, Matsuzawa D, Shimizu E. Oral administration of glycine increases extracellular serotonin but not dopamine in the prefrontal cortex of rats. *Psychiatry Clin Neurosci.* 2011;65(2):142-9.

174   Bannai M, Kawai N. New therapeutic strategy for amino acid medicine: glycine improves the quality of sleep. *J Pharmacol Sci.* 2012;118(2):145-8.

175   Kawai N, Sakai N, Okuro M, et al. The sleep-promoting and hypothermic effects of glycine are mediated by NMDA receptors in the suprachiasmatic nucleus. *Neuropsychopharmacology.* 2015;40(6):1405-16.

176   Melatonin for Treatment of Sleep Disorders. US Department of Health and Human Services website. http://archive.ahrq.gov/clinic/epcsums/melatsum.htm.

177   Banach M, Gurdziel E, Jędrych M, Borowicz KK. Melatonin in experimental seizures and epilepsy. *Pharmacol Rep.* 2011;63(1):1-11.

178   Melatonin for Treatment of Sleep Disorders. US Department of Health and Human Services website. http://archive.ahrq.gov/clinic/epcsums/melatsum.htm.

179   Melatonin Side Effects. Drugs.com website. http://www.drugs.com/sfx/melatonin-side-effects.html. Accessed 2009.

180   Dawson D, Gibbon S, Singh P. The hypothermic effect of melatonin on core body temperature: is more better? *J Pineal Res.* 1996 May;20(4):192-7.

181   Melatonin. Monograph. *Altern Med Rev.* 2005 Dec;10(4):326-36.

182   Melatonin for Treatment of Sleep Disorders. US Department of Health and Human Services website. http://archive.ahrq.gov/clinic/epcsums/melatsum.htm.

183   Melatonin for Treatment of Sleep Disorders. US Department of Health and Human Services website. http://archive.ahrq.gov/clinic/epcsums/melatsum.htm.

184   Andersen LP, Gögenur I, Rosenberg J, Reiter RJ. The Safety of Melatonin in Humans. *Clin Drug Investig.* 2016 Mar;36(3):169-75.

185   van Geijlswijk IM, Mol RH, Egberts TC, Smits MG. Evaluation of sleep, puberty and mental health in children with long-term melatonin treatment for chronic idiopathic childhood sleep onset insomnia. *Psychopharmacology (Berl).* 2011 Jul;216(1):111-20.

186   Lemoine P, Garfinkel D, Laudon M, Nir T, Zisapel N. Prolonged-release melatonin for insomnia - an open-label long-term study of efficacy, safety, and withdrawal. *Ther Clin Risk Manag.* 2011;7:301-11.

187   Lemoine P, Garfinkel D, Laudon M, Nir T, Zisapel N. Prolonged-release melatonin for insomnia - an open-label long-term study of efficacy, safety, and withdrawal. *Ther Clin Risk Manag.* 2011;7:301-11.

Notes

188   Lusardi P, Preti P, Savino S, Piazza E, Zoppi A, Fogari R. Effect of bedtime mela-tonin ingestion on blood pressure of normotensive subjects. *Blood Press Monit.* 1997 Apr;2(2):99-103.

189   Carrillo-Vico A, Lardone PJ, Alvarez-Sánchez N, Rodríguez-Rodríguez A, Guerrero JM. Melatonin: buffering the immune system. *Int J Mol Sci.* 2013 Apr 22;14(4):8638-83.

190   Maestroni GJ. The immunotherapeutic potential of melatonin. *Expert Opin Investig Drugs.* 2001 Mar;10(3):467-76.

191   Sutherland ER, Martin RJ, Ellison MC, Kraft M. Immunomodulatory effects of melatonin in asthma. *Am J Respir Crit Care Med.* 2002 Oct 15;166(8):1055-61.

192   Lemoine P, Garfinkel D, Laudon M, Nir T, Zisapel N. Prolonged-release melatonin for insomnia - an open-label long-term study of efficacy, safety, and withdrawal. *Ther Clin Risk Manag.* 2011;7:301-11.

193   Melatonin for Treatment of Sleep Disorders. US Department of Health and Human Services website. http://archive.ahrq.gov/clinic/epcsums/melatsum.htm.

194   Lemoine P, Garfinkel D, Laudon M, Nir T, Zisapel N. Prolonged-release melatonin for insomnia - an open-label long-term study of efficacy, safety, and withdrawal. *Ther Clin Risk Manag.* 2011;7:301-11.

195   Melatonin. University of Maryland Medical Center website. http://umm.edu/health/medical/altmed/supplement/melatonin. Reviewed February 3, 2016. Accessed May 24, 2016.

196   Van der Heijden KB, Smits MG, Van Someren EJ, Ridderinkhof KR, Gunning WB. Effect of melatonin on sleep, behavior, and cognition in ADHD and chronic sleep-onset insomnia. *J Am Acad Child Adolesc Psychiatry.* 2007 Feb;46(2):233-41.

197   Mostafavi SA, Mohammadi MR, Hosseinzadeh P, et al. Dietary intake, growth and development of children with ADHD in a randomized clinical trial of Ritalin and Mela-tonin co-administration: Through circadian cycle modification or appetite enhance-ment? *Iran J Psychiatry.* 2012 Summer;7(3):114-9.

198   Held K, Antonijevic IA, Künzel H, et al. Oral Mg(2+) supplementation reverses age-related neuroendocrine and sleep EEG changes in humans. *Pharmacopsychiatry.* 2002 Jul;35(4):135-43.

199   Hornyak M, Haas P, Veit J, Gann H, Riemann D. Magnesium treatment of primary alcohol-dependent patients during subacute withdrawal: an open pilot study with polysomnography. *Alcohol Clin Exp Res.* 2004 Nov;28(11):1702-9.

200   Tanabe K, Osada N, Suzuki N, et al. Erythrocyte magnesium and prostaglandin dynamics in chronic sleep deprivation. *Clin Cardiol.* 1997 Mar;20(3):265-8.

Chapter 11

201   Schuchardt JP, Huss M, Stauss-Grabo M, Hahn A. Significance of long chain poly-unsaturated fatty acids (PUFAs) for the development and behaviour of children. *Eur J Pediatr.* 2010 Feb;169(2):149-64.

202   Schuchardt JP, Huss M, Stauss-Grabo M, Hahn A. Significance of long-chain poly-unsaturated fatty acids (PUFAs) for the development and behaviour of children. *Eur J Pediatr.* 2010 Feb;169(2):149-64.

203   Schuchardt JP, Huss M, Stauss-Grabo M, Hahn A. Significance of long-chain poly-unsaturated fatty acids (PUFAs) for the development and behaviour of children. *Eur J Pediatr*. 2010 Feb;169(2):149-64.

204   Gow RV, Vallee-Tourangeau F, Crawford MA, et al. Omega-3 fatty acids are inverse-ly related to callous and unemotional traits in adolescent boys with attention deficit hyperactivity disorder. *Prostaglandins Leukot Essent Fatty Acids*. 2013;88(6):411-8.

205   Koletzko B, Demmelmair H, Schaeffer L, Illig T, Heinrich J. Genetically determined variation in polyunsaturated fatty acid metabolism may result in different dietary re-quirements. *Nestle Nutr Workshop Ser Pediatr Program*. 2008;62:35-44; discussion 44-9.

206   Brenna JT. Efficiency of conversion of alpha-linolenic acid to long chain n-3 fatty acids in man. *Curr Opin Clin Nutr Metab Care*. 2002 Mar;5(2):127-32.

207   Schuchardt JP, Huss M, Stauss-Grabo M, Hahn A. Significance of long-chain poly-unsaturated fatty acids (PUFAs) for the development and behaviour of children. *Eur J Pediatr*. 2010 Feb;169(2):149-64.

208   Brookes KJ, Chen W, Xu X, Taylor E, Asherson P. Association of fatty acid desat-urase genes with attention-deficit/hyperactivity disorder. *Biol Psychiatry*. 2006 Nov 15;60(10):1053-61.

209   Schuchardt JP, Huss M, Stauss-Grabo M, Hahn A. Significance of long-chain poly-unsaturated fatty acids (PUFAs) for the development and behaviour of children. *Eur J Pediatr*. 2010 Feb;169(2):149-64.

210   Schuchardt JP, Huss M, Stauss-Grabo M, Hahn A. Significance of long-chain poly-unsaturated fatty acids (PUFAs) for the development and behaviour of children. *Eur J Pediatr*. 2010 Feb;169(2):149-64.

211   Schuchardt JP, Huss M, Stauss-Grabo M, Hahn A. Significance of long-chain poly-unsaturated fatty acids (PUFAs) for the development and behaviour of children. *Eur J Pediatr*. 2010 Feb;169(2):149-64.

212   Hauswirth CB, Scheeder MR, Beer JH. High omega-3 fatty acid content in alpine cheese: the basis for an alpine paradox. *Circulation*. 2004 Jan 6;109(1):103-7.

213   Ross BM, McKenzie I, Glen I, Bennett CP. Increased levels of ethane, a non-in-vasive marker of n-3 fatty acid oxidation, in breath of children with attention deficit hyperactivity disorder. *Nutr Neurosci*. 2003 Oct;6(5):277-81.

214   Chalon S, Delion-Vancassel S, Belzung C, et al. Dietary fish oil affects monoami-nergic neurotransmission and behavior in rats. *J Nutr*. 1998 Dec;128(12):2512-9.

215   Hirayama S, Masuda Y, Rabeler R. Effect of phosphatidylserine administration on symptoms of attention-deficit/hyperactivity disorder in children. *Agro Food*. 2006;17(5):32-36.

216   Delion S, Chalon S, Guilloteau D, Lejeune B, Besnard JC, Durand G. Age-related changes in phospholipid fatty acid composition and monoaminergic neurotrans-mission in the hippocampus of rats fed a balanced or an n-3 polyunsaturated fatty acid-deficient diet. *J Lipid Res*. 1997 Apr;38(4):680-9.

217   Bloch MH, Qawasmi A. Omega-3 fatty acid supplementation for the treatment of children with attention-deficit/hyperactivity disorder symptomatology: systematic review and meta-analysis. *J Am Acad Child Adolesc Psychiatry*. 2011 Oct;50(10):991-1000.

Notes

218   Puri BK, Martins JG. Which polyunsaturated fatty acids are active in children with attention-deficit hyperactivity disorder receiving PUFA supplementation? A fatty acid validated meta-regression analysis of randomized controlled trials. *Prostaglandins Leukot Essent Fatty Acids.* 2014;90(5):179-89.

219   Milte CM, Parletta N, Buckley JD, Coates AM, Young RM, Howe PR. Increased erythrocyte eicosapentaenoic acid and docosahexaenoic acid are associated with improved attention and behavior in children with ADHD in a randomized controlled three-way crossover trial. *J Atten Disord.* 2015;19(11):954-64.

220   Cisár P, Jány R, Waczulíková I, et al. Effect of pine bark extract (Pycnogenol) on symptoms of knee osteoarthritis. *Phytother Res.* 2008 Aug;22(8):1087-92.

221   Sorgi PJ, Hallowell EM, Hutchins HL, Sears B. Effects of an open-label pilot study with high-dose EPA/DHA concentrates on plasma phospholipids and behavior in children with attention deficit hyperactivity disorder. *Nutr J.* 2007 Jul 13;6:16.

222   Gustafsson PA, Birberg-Thornberg U, Duchén K, et al. EPA supplementation improves teacher-rated behaviour and oppositional symptoms in children with ADHD. *Acta Paediatr.* 2010 Oct;99(10):1540-9. doi: 10.1111/j.1651-2227.2010.01871.x.

223   Lorente-Cebrián S, Costa AG, Navas-Carretero S, Zabala M, Martínez JA, Moreno-Aliaga MJ. Role of omega-3 fatty acids in obesity, metabolic syndrome, and cardiovascular diseases: a review of the evidence. *J Physiol Biochem.* 2013 Sep;69(3):633-51. doi: 10.1007/s13105-013-0265-4.

224   Rangel-Huerta OD, Aguilera CM, Mesa MD, Gil A. Omega-3 long-chain polyunsaturated fatty acids supplementation on inflammatory biomakers: a systematic review of randomised clinical trials. *Br J Nutr.* 2012 Jun;107 Suppl 2:S159-70. doi: 10.1017/S0007114512001559.

225   Peter S, Chopra S, Jacob JJ. A fish a day, keeps the cardiologist away! - A review of the effect of omega-3 fatty acids in the cardiovascular system. *Indian J Endocrinol Metab.* 2013 May;17(3):422-9. doi: 10.4103/2230-8210.111630.

226   Zhang M, Picard-Deland E, Marette A. Fish and Marine Omega-3 Polyunsatured Fatty Acid Consumption and Incidence of Type 2 Diabetes: A Systematic Review and Meta-Analysis. *Int J Endocrinol.* 2013;2013:501015.

227   Parker HM, Johnson NA, Burdon CA, Cohn JS, O'Connor HT, George J. Omega-3 supplementation and non-alcoholic fatty liver disease: a systematic review and meta-analysis. *J Hepatol.* 2012 Apr;56(4):944-51. doi: 10.1016/j.jhep.2011.08.018.

228   Lorente-Cebrián S, Costa AG, Navas-Carretero S, Zabala M, Martínez JA, Moreno-Aliaga MJ. Role of omega-3 fatty acids in obesity, metabolic syndrome, and cardiovascular diseases: a review of the evidence. *J Physiol Biochem.* 2013 Sep;69(3):633-51. doi: 10.1007/s13105-013-0265-4.

229   Miles EA, Calder PC. Influence of marine n-3 polyunsaturated fatty acids on immune function and a systematic review of their effects on clinical outcomes in rheumatoid arthritis. *Br J Nutr.* 2012 Jun;107 Suppl 2:S171-84. doi: 10.1017/S0007114512001560.

230   Vines A, Delattre AM, Lima MM, et al. The role of 5-HT$_1$A receptors in fish oil-mediated increased BDNF expression in the rat hippocampus and cortex: a possible antidepressant mechanism. *Neuropharmacology.* 2012 Jan;62(1):184-91. doi: 10.1016/j.neuropharm.2011.06.017.

231   Bloch MH, Hannestad J. Omega-3 fatty acids for the treatment of depression: systematic review and meta-analysis. *Mol Psychiatry.* 2012 Dec;17(12):1272-82. doi: 10.1038/mp.2011.100.

232   Balanzá-Martínez V, Fries GR, Colpo GD, et al. Therapeutic use of omega-3 fatty acids in bipolar disorder. *Expert Rev Neurother.* 2011 Jul;11(7):1029-47. doi: 10.1586/ ern.11.42.

233   Bent S, Bertoglio K, Hendren RL. Omega-3 fatty acids for autistic spectrum disorder: a systematic review. *J Autism Dev Disord.* 2009 Aug;39(8):1145-54. doi: 10.1007/ s10803-009-0724-5.

234   Van der Kemp WJ, Klomp DW, Kahn RS, Luijten PR, Hulshoff Pol HE. A meta-analysis of the polyunsaturated fatty acid composition of erythrocyte membranes in schizophrenia. *Schizophr Res.* 2012 Nov;141(2-3):153-61. doi: 10.1016/j.schres.2012.08.014.

235   Fusar-Poli P, Berger G. Eicosapentaenoic acid interventions in schizophrenia: meta-analysis of randomized, placebo-controlled studies. *J Clin Psychopharmacol.* 2012 Apr;32(2):179-85. doi: 10.1097/JCP.0b013e318248b7bb.

236   Mossaheb N, Schloegelhofer M, Schaefer MR, et al. Polyunsaturated fatty acids in emerging psychosis. *Curr Pharm Des.* 2012;18(4):576-91.

237   Kozielec T, Starobrat-Hermelin B. Assessment of magnesium levels in children with attention deficit hyperactivity disorder (ADHD). *Magnes Res.* 1997 Jun;10(2):143-8.

238   Zanarini MC, Frankenburg FR. omega-3 Fatty acid treatment of women with borderline personality disorder: a double-blind, placebo-controlled pilot study. *Am J Psychiatry.* 2003 Jan;160(1):167-9.

239   Lindmark L, Clough P. A 5-month open study with long-chain polyunsaturated fatty acids in dyslexia. *J Med Food.* 2007 Dec;10(4):662-6.

240   Long SJ, Benton D. A double-blind trial of the effect of docosahexaenoic acid and vitamin and mineral supplementation on aggression, impulsivity, and stress. *Hum Psychopharmacol.* 2013 May;28(3):238-47. doi: 10.1002/hup.2313.

241   Loef M, Walach H. The omega-6/omega-3 ratio and dementia or cognitive decline: a systematic review on human studies and biological evidence. *J Nutr Gerontol Geriatr.* 2013;32(1):1-23. doi: 10.1080/21551197.2012.752335.

242   Puri BK, Martins JG. Which polyunsaturated fatty acids are active in children with attention-deficit hyperactivity disorder receiving PUFA supplementation? A fatty acid validated meta-regression analysis of randomized controlled trials. *Prostaglandins Leukot Essent Fatty Acids.* 2014;90(5):179-89.

243   GRAS Notices. GRN No. 394. Dried biomass of *Arthrospira platensis*, also known as Spirulina platensis (Spirulina). U.S. Food and Drug Administration website. http://www. accessdata.fda.gov/scripts/fdcc/index.cfm?set=GRASNotices&id=394. Updated October 30, 2015.

244   GRAS Notices. GRN No. 486. Oil from the seeds of *Buglossoides arvensis*. U.S. Food and Drug Administration website. http://www.accessdata.fda.gov/scripts/fdcc/index. cfm?set=GRASNotices&id=486. Updated October 30, 2015.

245   University of Maryland Medical Center website. Gamma-linolenic acid. http://umm. edu/health/medical/altmed/supplement/gammalinolenic-acid. Updated June 24, 2013.

Notes

246 Puri BK. The safety of evening primrose oil in epilepsy. *Prostaglandins Leukot Essent Fatty Acids*. 2007;77(2):101-3.

247 University of Maryland Medical Center website. Gamma-linolenic acid. http://umm.edu/health/medical/altmed/supplement/gammalinolenic-acid. Updated June 24, 2013.

248 University of Maryland Medical Center website. Gamma-linolenic acid. http://umm.edu/health/medical/altmed/supplement/gammalinolenic-acid. Updated June 24, 2013.

249 University of Maryland Medical Center website. Gamma-linolenic acid. http://umm.edu/health/medical/altmed/supplement/gammalinolenic-acid. Updated June 24, 2013.

250 University of Maryland Medical Center website. Gamma-linolenic acid. http://umm.edu/health/medical/altmed/supplement/gammalinolenic-acid. Updated June 24, 2013.

251 Manor I, Ben-Hayun R, Aharon-Peretz J, et al. A randomized, double-blind, placebo-controlled, multicenter study evaluating the efficacy, safety, and tolerability of extended-release metadoxine in adults with attention-deficit/hyperactivity disorder. *J Clin Psychiatry*. 2012;73(12):1517-23.

252 Kozielec T, Starobrat-Hermelin B. Assessment of magnesium levels in children with attention deficit hyperactivity disorder (ADHD). *Magnes Res*. 1997 Jun;10(2):143-8.

253 Starobrat-Hermelin B, Kozielec T. The effects of magnesium physiological supplementation on hyperactivity in children with attention deficit hyperactivity disorder (ADHD). Positive response to magnesium oral loading test. *Magnes Res*. 1997 Jun;10(2):149-56.

254 Mousain-Bosc M, Roche M, Polge A, Pradal-Prat D, Rapin J, Bali JP. Improvement of neurobehavioral disorders in children supplemented with magnesium-vitamin B6. I. Attention deficit hyperactivity disorders. *Magnes Res*. 2006 Mar;19(1):46-52.

255 Poleszak E. Modulation of antidepressant-like activity of magnesium by serotonergic system. *Neural Transm*. 2007 Sep;114(9):1129-34.

256 Mousain-Bosc M, Roche M, Rapin J, Bali JP. Magnesium VitB6 intake reduces central nervous system hyperexcitability in children. *J Am Coll Nutr*. 2004 Oct;23(5):545S-548S.

257 Mousain-Bosc M, Roche M, Rapin J, Bali JP. Magnesium VitB6 intake reduces central nervous system hyperexcitability in children. *J Am Coll Nutr*. 2004 Oct;23(5):545S-548S.

258 Starobrat-Hermelin B, Kozielec T. The effects of magnesium physiological supplementation on hyperactivity in children with attention deficit hyperactivity disorder (ADHD). Positive response to magnesium oral loading test. *Magnes Res*. 1997 Jun;10(2):149-56.

259 Dolina S, Margalit D, Malitsky S, Rabinkov A. Attention-deficit hyperactivity disorder (ADHD) as a pyridoxine-dependent condition: urinary diagnostic biomarkers. *Med Hypotheses*. 2014;82(1):111-6.

260 Dolina S, Margalit D, Malitsky S, Rabinkov A. Attention-deficit hyperactivity disorder (ADHD) as a pyridoxine-dependent condition: urinary diagnostic biomarkers. *Med Hypotheses*. 2014;82(1):111-6.

261 Guerrini I, Gentili C, Nelli G, Guazzelli M. A follow up study on the efficacy of metadoxine in the treatment of alcohol dependence. *Subst Abuse Treat Prev Policy*. 2006;1:35.

262   Manor I, Ben-Hayun R, Aharon-Peretz J, et al. A randomized, double-blind, placebo-controlled, multicenter study evaluating the efficacy, safety, and tolerability of extended-release metadoxine in adults with attention-deficit/hyperactivity disorder. *J Clin Psychiatry*. 2012;73(12):1517-23.

263   Manor I, Ben-Hayun R, Aharon-Peretz J, et al. A randomized, double-blind, placebo-controlled, multicenter study evaluating the efficacy, safety, and tolerability of extended-release metadoxine in adults with attention-deficit/hyperactivity disorder. *J Clin Psychiatry*. 2012;73(12):1517-23.

264   Manor I, Rubin J, Daniely Y, Adler LA. Attention benefits after a single dose of metadoxine extended release in adults with predominantly inattentive ADHD. *Postgrad Med*. 2014;126(5):7-16.

265   Manor I, Ben-Hayun R, Aharon-Peretz J, et al. A randomized, double-blind, placebo-controlled, multicenter study evaluating the efficacy, safety, and tolerability of extended-release metadoxine in adults with attention-deficit/hyperactivity disorder. *J Clin Psychiatry*. 2012;73(12):1517-23.

266   Manor I, Newcorn JH, Faraone SV, Adler LA. Efficacy of metadoxine extended release in patients with predominantly inattentive subtype attention-deficit/hyperactivity disorder. *Postgrad Med*. 2013;125(4):181-90.

267   Fornai F, Grazia Alessandrì M, Bonuccelli U, Scalori V, Corsini GU. Effect of metadoxine on striatal dopamine levels in C57 black mice. *J Pharm Pharmacol*. 1993;45(5):476-8.

268   Antonelli T, Carlà V, Lambertini L, Moroni F, Bianchi C. Pyroglutamic acid administration modifies the electrocorticogram and increases the release of acetylcholine and GABA from the guinea-pig cerebral cortex. *Pharmacol Res Commun*. 1984;16(2):189-97.

269   Koletzko B, Demmelmair H, Schaeffer L, Illig T, Heinrich J. Genetically determined variation in polyunsaturated fatty acid metabolism may result in different dietary requirements. *Nestle Nutr Workshop Ser Pediatr Program*. 2008;62:35-44; discussion 44-9.

270   Poleszak E. Modulation of antidepressant-like activity of magnesium by serotonergic system. *Neural Transm*. 2007 Sep;114(9):1129-34.

271   Koletzko B, Demmelmair H, Schaeffer L, Illig T, Heinrich J. Genetically determined variation in polyunsaturated fatty acid metabolism may result in different dietary requirements. *Nestle Nutr Workshop Ser Pediatr Program*. 2008;62:35-44; discussion 44-9.

272   Mousain-Bosc M, Roche M, Rapin J, Bali JP. Magnesium VitB6 intake reduces central nervous system hyperexcitability in children. *J Am Coll Nutr*. 2004 Oct;23(5):545S-548S.

273   Vitamin B6 (pyridoxine and pyridoxal 5'-phosphate) - monograph. *Altern Med Rev*. 2001 Feb;6(1):87-92.

274   Vitamin B6 (pyridoxine and pyridoxal 5'-phosphate) - monograph. *Altern Med Rev*. 2001 Feb;6(1):87-92.

275   Vitamin B6 (pyridoxine and pyridoxal 5'-phosphate) - monograph. *Altern Med Rev*. 2001 Feb;6(1):87-92.

276   Eby GA, Eby KL. Rapid recovery from major depression using magnesium treatment. *Med Hypotheses*. 2006;67(2):362-70.

Notes

277   Kiddie JY, Weiss MD, Kitts DD, Levy-Milne R, Wasdell MB. Nutritional status of children with attention deficit hyperactivity disorder: a pilot study. *Int J Pediatr.* 2010;2010:767318.

278   Krause J. SPECT and PET of the dopamine transporter in attention-deficit/hyperactivity disorder. *Expert Rev Neurother.* 2008 Apr;8(4):611-25.

279   Arnold LE, Disilvestro RA, Bozzolo D, et al. Zinc for attention-deficit/hyperactivity disorder: placebo-controlled double-blind pilot trial alone and combined with amphetamine. *J Child Adolesc Psychopharmacol.* 2011 Feb;21(1):1-19.

280   Dodig-Curković K, Dovhanj J, Curković M, Dodig-Radić J, Degmecić D. The role of zinc in the treatment of hyperactivity disorder in children. *Acta Med Croatica.* 2009 Oct;63(4):307-13.

281   Kiddie JY, Weiss MD, Kitts DD, Levy-Milne R, Wasdell MB. Nutritional status of children with attention deficit hyperactivity disorder: a pilot study. *Int J Pediatr.* 2010;2010:767318.

282   Lepping P, Huber M. Role of zinc in the pathogenesis of attention-deficit hyperactivity disorder: implications for research and treatment. *CNS Drugs.* 2010 Sep 1;24(9):721-8. doi: 10.2165/11537610-000000000-00000.

283   Donfrancesco R, Parisi P, Vanacore N, Martines F, Sargentini V, Cortese S. Iron and ADHD: time to move beyond serum ferritin levels. *J Atten Disord.* 2013;17(4):347-57.

284   Donfrancesco R, Parisi P, Vanacore N, Martines F, Sargentini V, Cortese S. Iron and ADHD: time to move beyond serum ferritin levels. *J Atten Disord.* 2013;17(4):347-57.

285   Arnold LE, Disilvestro RA, Bozzolo D, et al. Zinc for attention-deficit/hyperactivity disorder: placebo-controlled double-blind pilot trial alone and combined with amphetamine. *J Child Adolesc Psychopharmacol.* 2011;21(1):1-19.

286   Tan LN, Wei HY, Zhang YD, Lu AL, Li Y. Relationship between serum ferritin levels and susceptibility to attention deficit hyperactivity disorder in children: a meta analysis [in Chinese]. *Zhongguo Dang Dai Er Ke Za Zhi.* 2011;13(9):722-4.

287   Oner O, Oner P, Bozkurt OH, et al. Effects of zinc and ferritin levels on parent and teacher reported symptom scores in attention deficit hyperactivity disorder. *Child Psychiatry Hum Dev.* 2010;41(4):441-7.

288   Calarge C, Farmer C, DiSilvestro R, Arnold LE. Serum ferritin and amphetamine response in youth with attention-deficit/hyperactivity disorder. *J Child Adolesc Psychopharmacol.* 2010;20(6):495-502.

289   Lahat E, Heyman E, Livne A, Goldman M, Berkovitch M, Zachor D. Iron deficiency in children with attention deficit hyperactivity disorder. *Isr Med Assoc J.* 2011;13(9):530-3.

290   Oner O, Alkar OY, Oner P. Relation of ferritin levels with symptom ratings and cognitive performance in children with attention deficit-hyperactivity disorder. *Pediatr Int.* 2008;50(1):40-4.

291   Oner O, Alkar OY, Oner P. Relation of ferritin levels with symptom ratings and cognitive performance in children with attention deficit-hyperactivity disorder. *Pediatr Int.* 2008;50(1):40-4.

292   Oner O, Oner P, Bozkurt OH, et al. Effects of zinc and ferritin levels on parent and teacher reported symptom scores in attention deficit hyperactivity disorder. *Child Psychiatry Hum Dev.* 2010;41(4):441-7.

293   Soto-Insuga V, Calleja ML, Prados M, Castaño C, Losada R, Ruiz-Falcó ML. Role of iron in the treatment of attention deficit-hyperactivity disorder [in Spanish]. *An Pediatr (Barc)*. 2013;79(4):230-5.

294   Abou-Khadra MK, Amin OR, Shaker OG, Rabah TM. Parent-reported sleep problems, symptom ratings, and serum ferritin levels in children with attention-deficit/hyperactivity disorder: a case control study. *BMC Pediatr*. 2013;13:217.

295   Lahat E, Heyman E, Livne A, Goldman M, Berkovitch M, Zachor D. Iron deficiency in children with attention deficit hyperactivity disorder. *Isr Med Assoc J*. 2011;13(9):530-3.

296   Calarge C, Farmer C, DiSilvestro R, Arnold LE. Serum ferritin and amphetamine response in youth with attention-deficit/hyperactivity disorder. *J Child Adolesc Psychopharmacol*. 2010;20(6):495-502.

297   Oner O, Oner P, Bozkurt OH, et al. Effects of zinc and ferritin levels on parent and teacher reported symptom scores in attention deficit hyperactivity disorder. *Child Psychiatry Hum Dev*. 2010;41(4):441-7.

298   Bener A, Kamal M, Bener H, Bhugra D. Higher prevalence of iron deficiency as strong predictor of attention deficit hyperactivity disorder in children. *Ann Med Health Sci Res*. 2014;4(suppl 3):S291-7.

299   Goksugur SB, Tufan AE, Semiz M, et al. Vitamin D status in children with attention-deficit-hyperactivity disorder. *Pediatr Int*. 2014;56(4):515-9.

300   Bener A, Kamal M. Predict attention deficit hyperactivity disorder? Evidence-based medicine. *Glob J Health Sci*. 2013;6(2):47-57.

301   McCann JC, Ames BN. Is there convincing biological or behavioral evidence linking vitamin D deficiency to brain dysfunction? *FASEB J*. 2008 Apr;22(4):982-1001.

302   McCann JC, Ames BN. Is there convincing biological or behavioral evidence linking vitamin D deficiency to brain dysfunction? *FASEB J*. 2008 Apr;22(4):982-1001.

303   Holick MF. Resurrection of vitamin D deficiency and rickets. J Clin Invest. 2006 Aug;116(8):2062-72.

304   Holick MF. Resurrection of vitamin D deficiency and rickets. *J Clin Invest*. 2006 Aug;116(8):2062-72.

305   National Institutes of Health. Vitamin D Fact Sheet for Health Professionals. https://ods.od.nih.gov/factsheets/VitaminD-HealthProfessional/ Updated February 11, 2016.

306   Forsythe P, Sudo N, Dinan T, Taylor VH, Bienenstock J. Mood and gut feelings. *Brain Behav Immun*. 2010 Jan;24(1):9-16. doi: 10.1016/j.bbi.2009.05.058. Epub 2009 May 28.

307   Forsythe P, Sudo N, Dinan T, Taylor VH, Bienenstock J. Mood and gut feelings. *Brain Behav Immun*. 2010 Jan;24(1):9-16. doi: 10.1016/j.bbi.2009.05.058. Epub 2009 May 28.

308   Nogueira JC, Gonçalves Mda C. Probiotics in allergic rhinitis. *Braz J Otorhinolaryngol*. 2011 Jan-Feb;77(1):129-34.

309   Frei R, Lauener RP, Crameri R, O'Mahony L. Microbiota and dietary interactions: an update to the hygiene hypothesis? *Allergy*. 2012 Apr;67(4):451-61. doi: 10.1111/j.1398-9995.2011.02783.x.

Notes

310   Ozdemir O. Various effects of different probiotic strains in allergic disorders: an update from laboratory and clinical data. *Clin Exp Immunol.* 2010 Jun;160(3):295-304.

311   Ozdemir O. Various effects of different probiotic strains in allergic disorders: an update from laboratory and clinical data. *Clin Exp Immunol.* 2010 Jun;160(3):295-304.

312   Ozdemir O. Various effects of different probiotic strains in allergic disorders: an update from laboratory and clinical data. *Clin Exp Immunol.* 2010 Jun;160(3):295-304.

313   Ozdemir O. Various effects of different probiotic strains in allergic disorders: an update from laboratory and clinical data. *Clin Exp Immunol.* 2010 Jun;160(3):295-304.

314   Ozdemir O. Various effects of different probiotic strains in allergic disorders: an update from laboratory and clinical data. *Clin Exp Immunol.* 2010 Jun;160(3):295-304.

315   Frei R, Lauener RP, Crameri R, O'Mahony L. Microbiota and dietary interactions: an update to the hygiene hypothesis? *Allergy.* 2012 Apr;67(4):451-61. doi: 10.1111/j.1398-9995.2011.02783.x.

316   Naidu KSB, Adam JK, Govender P. The use of probiotics and safety concerns: a review. *Afr J Microbiol* Res. 2012;6(41):6871-77. http://www.academicjournals.org/article/article1380538370_Naidu%20et%20al.pdf.

317   Critchfield JW, van Hemert S, Ash M, Mulder L, Ashwood P. The potential role of probiotics in the management of childhood autism spectrum disorders. *Gastroenterol Res Pract.* 2011;2011:161358.

318   Guarner F, Requena T, Marcos A. Consensus statements from the Workshop "Probiotics and Health: Scientific evidence." *Nutr Hosp.* 2010 Sep-Oct;25(5):700-4.

319   Ozdemir O. Any benefits of probiotics in allergic disorders? *Allergy Asthma Proc.* 2010 Mar-Apr;31(2):103-11.

320   Del Giudice MM, Leonardi S, Maiello N, Brunese FP. Food allergy and probiotics in childhood. *J Clin Gastroenterol.* 2010 Sep;44 Suppl 1:S22-5.

321   Raison CL, Lowry CA, Rook GA. Inflammation, sanitation, and consternation: loss of contact with coevolved, tolerogenic microorganisms and the pathophysiology and treatment of major depression. *Arch Gen Psychiatry.* 2010 Dec;67(12):1211-24.

322   Raison CL, Lowry CA, Rook GA. Inflammation, sanitation, and consternation: loss of contact with coevolved, tolerogenic microorganisms and the pathophysiology and treatment of major depression. *Arch Gen Psychiatry.* 2010 Dec;67(12):1211-24.

323   Gill H, Prasad J. Probiotics, immunomodulation, and health benefits. *Adv Exp Med Biol.* 2008;606:423-54.

324   Adams JB, Johansen LJ, Powell LD, Quig D, Rubin RA. Gastrointestinal flora and gastrointestinal status in children with autism--comparisons to typical children and correlation with autism severity. *BMC Gastroenterol.* 2011 Mar 16;11:22.

325   Logan AC, Katzman M. Major depressive disorder: probiotics may be an adjuvant therapy. *Med Hypotheses.* 2005;64(3):533-8.

326   Bercik P, Verdu EF, Foster JA, et al. Chronic gastrointestinal inflammation induces anxiety-like behavior and alters central nervous system biochemistry in mice. *Gastroenterology.* 2010 Dec;139(6):2102-2112.e1.

327   Diop L, Guillou S, Durand H. Probiotic food supplement reduces stress-induced gastrointestinal symptoms in volunteers: a double-blind, placebo-controlled, randomized trial. *Nutr Res.* 2008 Jan;28(1):1-5.

328   Bravo JA, Forsythe P, Chew MV, et al. Ingestion of Lactobacillus strain regulates emotional behavior and central GABA receptor expression in a mouse via the vagus nerve. *Proc Natl Acad Sci U S A.* 2011;108(38):16050-16055. doi

329   Markus CR, Jonkman LM, Lammers JH, Deutz NE, Messer MH, Rigtering N. Evening intake of alpha-lactalbumin increases plasma tryptophan availability and improves morning alertness and brain measures of attention. *Am J Clin Nutr.* 2005 May;81(5):1026-33.

330   Lutgendorff F, Akkermans LM, Söderholm JD. The role of microbiota and probiotics in stress-induced gastro-intestinal damage. *Curr Mol Med.* 2008 Jun;8(4):282-98.

331   Marcos A, Wärnberg J, Nova E, et al. The effect of milk fermented by yogurt cultures plus Lactobacillus casei DN-114001 on the immune response of subjects under academic examination stress. *Eur J Nutr.* 2004 Dec;43(6):381-9.

332   Gareau MG, Jury J, MacQueen G, Sherman PM, Perdue MH. Probiotic treatment of rat pups normalises corticosterone release and ameliorates colonic dysfunction induced by maternal separation. *Gut.* 2007 Nov;56(11):1522-8. Epub 2007 Mar 5.

333   Lyon MR. *Is Your Child's Brain Starving?* Coquitlam, British Columbia, Canada: Mind Publishing; 2002.

334   Chovanová Z, Muchová J, Sivonová M, et al. Effect of polyphenolic extract, Pycnogenol, on the level of 8-oxoguanine in children suffering from attention deficit/hyperactivity disorder. *Free Radic Res.* 2006 Sep;40(9):1003-10.

335   Chovanová Z, Muchová J, Sivonová M, et al. Effect of polyphenolic extract, Pycnogenol, on the level of 8-oxoguanine in children suffering from attention deficit/hyperactivity disorder. *Free Radic Res.* 2006 Sep;40(9):1003-10.

336   Lutgendorff F, Trulsson LM, van Minnen LP, et al. Probiotics enhance pancreatic glutathione biosynthesis and reduce oxidative stress in experimental acute pancreatitis. *Am J Physiol Gastrointest Liver Physiol.* 2008 Nov;295(5):G1111-21.

337   Asemi Z, Jazayeri S, Najafi M, et al. Effect of daily consumption of probiotic yogurt on oxidative stress in pregnant women: a randomized controlled clinical trial. *Ann Nutr Metab.* 2012;60(1):62-8.

338   Ejtahed HS, Mohtadi-Nia J, Homayouni-Rad A, Niafar M, Asghari-Jafarabadi M, Mofid V. Probiotic yogurt improves antioxidant status in type 2 diabetic patients. *Nutrition.* 2012 May;28(5):539-43.

339   Bulut M, Selek S, Gergerlioglu HS, et al. Malondialdehyde levels in adult attention-deficit hyperactivity disorder. *J Psychiatry Neurosci.* 2007 Nov;32(6):435-8.

340   Nardone G, Compare D, Liguori E, et al. Protective effects of Lactobacillus paracasei F19 in a rat model of oxidative and metabolic hepatic injury. *Am J Physiol Gastrointest Liver Physiol.* 2010 Sep;299(3):G669-76.

341   Martarelli D, Verdenelli MC, Scuri S, et al. Effect of a probiotic intake on oxidant and antioxidant parameters in plasma of athletes during intense exercise training. *Curr Microbiol.* 2011 Jun;62(6):1689-96.

342   Martarelli D, Verdenelli MC, Scuri S, et al. Effect of a probiotic intake on oxidant and antioxidant parameters in plasma of athletes during intense exercise training. *Curr Microbiol.* 2011 Jun;62(6):1689-96.

Notes

343   Aldinucci C, Bellussi L, Monciatti G, et al. Effects of dietary yoghurt on immunological and clinical parameters of rhinopathic patients. *Eur J Clin Nutr.* 2002 Dec;56(12):1155-61.

344   Lin TY, Chen CJ, Chen LK, Wen SH, Jan RH. Effect of probiotics on allergic rhinitis in Df, Dp or dust-sensitive children: a randomized double blind controlled trial. *Indian Pediatr.* 2013;50(2):209-13.

345   Giovannini M, Agostoni C, Riva E, et al. A randomized prospective double blind controlled trial on effects of long-term consumption of fermented milk containing Lactobacillus casei in pre-school children with allergic asthma and/or rhinitis. *Pediatr Res.* 2007 Aug;62(2):215-20.

346   Chen YS, Jan RL, Lin YL, Chen HH, Wang JY. Randomized placebo-controlled trial of lactobacillus on asthmatic children with allergic rhinitis. *Pediatr Pulmonol.* 2010 Nov;45(11):1111-20.

347   Wassenberg J, Nutten S, Audran R, et al. Effect of Lactobacillus paracasei ST11 on a nasal provocation test with grass pollen in allergic rhinitis. *Clin Exp Allergy.* 2011 Apr;41(4):565-73. doi: 10.1111/j.1365-2222.2011.03695.x.

348   Nagata Y, Yoshida M, Kitazawa H, Araki E, Gomyo T. Improvements in seasonal allergic disease with Lactobacillus plantarum No. 14. *Biosci Biotechnol Biochem.* 2010;74(9):1869-77.

349   Lin TY, Chen CJ, Chen LK, Wen SH, Jan RH. Effect of probiotics on allergic rhinitis in Df, Dp or dust-sensitive children: a randomized double blind controlled trial. *Indian Pediatr.* 2013;50(2):209-13.

350   Lin TY, Chen CJ, Chen LK, Wen SH, Jan RH. Effect of probiotics on allergic rhinitis in Df, Dp or dust-sensitive children: a randomized double blind controlled trial. *Indian Pediatr.* 2013;50(2):209-13.

351   Lin TY, Chen CJ, Chen LK, Wen SH, Jan RH. Effect of probiotics on allergic rhinitis in Df, Dp or dust-sensitive children: a randomized double blind controlled trial. *Indian Pediatr.* 2013;50(2):209-13.

352   Xiao JZ, Kondo S, Yanagisawa N, et al. Probiotics in the treatment of Japanese cedar pollinosis: a double-blind placebo-controlled trial. *Clin Exp Allergy.* 2006 Nov;36(11):1425-35.

353   Vliagoftis H, Kouranos VD, Betsi GI, Falagas ME. Probiotics for the treatment of allergic rhinitis and asthma: systematic review of randomized controlled trials. *Ann Allergy Asthma Immunol.* 2008 Dec;101(6):570-9.

354   Bercik P, Verdu EF, Foster JA, et al. Chronic gastrointestinal inflammation induces anxiety-like behavior and alters central nervous system biochemistry in mice. *Gastroenterology.* 2010 Dec;139(6):2102-2112.e1.

355   Kim JY, Choi YO, Ji GE. Effect of oral probiotics (Bifidobacterium lactis AD011 and Lactobacillus acidophilus AD031) administration on ovalbumin-induced food allergy mouse model. *J Microbiol Biotechnol.* 2008 Aug;18(8):1393-400.

356   Zhang LL, Chen X, Zheng PY, et al. Oral Bifidobacterium modulates intestinal immune inflammation in mice with food allergy. *J Gastroenterol Hepatol.* 2010 May;25(5):928-34.

357   Zuercher AW, Weiss M, Holvoet S, et al. Lactococcus lactis NCC 2287 alleviates food allergic manifestations in sensitized mice by reducing IL-13 expression specifically in the ileum. *Clin Dev Immunol.* 2012;2012:485750.

358   VSL#3 website. http://www.vsl3.com/hcp/vsl-info/. Accessed 2016.

359   Naidu KSB, Adam JK, Govender P. The use of probiotics and safety concerns: a review. *Afr J Microbiol Res.* 2012;6(41):6871-77. http://www.academicjournals.org/article/article1380538370_Naidu%20et%20al.pdf.

360   Jones K. Probiotics: preventing antibiotic-associated diarrhea. *J Spec Pediatr Nurs.* 2010 Apr;15(2):160-2. doi: 10.1111/j.1744-6155.2010.00231.x.

361   Introduction of a Qualified Presumption of Safety (QPS) approach for assessment of selected microorganisms referred to EFSA. European Food Safety Authority website. http://www.efsa.europa.eu/sites/default/files/scientific_output/files/main_documents/sc_op_ej587_qps_en%2C3.pdf. Accessed 2010.

362   Popova M, Molimard P, Courau S, et al. Beneficial effects of probiotics in upper respiratory tract infections and their mechanical actions to antagonize pathogens. *J Appl Microbiol.* 2012 Dec;113(6):1305-18. doi: 10.1111/j.1365-2672.2012.05394.x.

363   Mattia A, Merker R. Regulation of Probiotic Substances as Ingredients in Foods: Premarket Approval or "Generally Recognized as Safe" Notification. *Clin Infect Dis.* 2008;46(suppl 2):S115-8. http://cid.oxfordjournals.org/content/46/Supplement_2/S115.long. Accessed 2010.

364   Safety of Probiotics to Reduce Risk and Prevent or Treat Disease. Agency for Healthcare Research and Quality, U.S. Department of Health and Human Services website. http://www.ahrq.gov/downloads/pub/evidence/pdf/probiotics/probiotics.pdf. Updated April 2001.

365   Naidu KSB, Adam JK, Govender P. The use of probiotics and safety concerns: a review. *Afr J Microbiol Res.* 2012;6(41):6871-77. http://www.academicjournals.org/article/article1380538370_Naidu%20et%20al.pdf.

366   Hempel S, Newberry S, Ruelaz A, Wang Z, Miles JN, Suttorp MJ, Johnsen B, Shanman R, Slusser W, Fu N, Smith A, Roth B, Polak J, Motala A, Perry T, Shekelle PG. Safety of probiotics used to reduce risk and prevent or treat disease. Evid Rep Technol Assess (Full Rep). 2011 Apr;(200):1-645.

367   Rucklidge JJ, Johnstone J, Kaplan BJ. Nutrient supplementation approaches in the treatment of ADHD. *Expert Rev Neurother.* 2009 Apr;9(4):461-76. doi: 10.1586/ern.09.7.

368   Rucklidge JJ, Johnstone J, Kaplan BJ. Nutrient supplementation approaches in the treatment of ADHD. *Expert Rev Neurother.* 2009 Apr;9(4):461-76. doi: 10.1586/ern.09.7.

369   Rucklidge JJ, Johnstone J, Kaplan BJ. Nutrient supplementation approaches in the treatment of ADHD. *Expert Rev Neurother.* 2009 Apr;9(4):461-76. doi: 10.1586/ern.09.7.

370   Harding KL, Judah RD, Gant C. Outcome-based comparison of Ritalin versus food-supplement treated children with AD/HD. *Altern Med Rev.* 2003 Aug;8(3):319-30.

371   Huss M, Völp A, Stauss-Grabo M. Supplementation of polyunsaturated fatty acids, magnesium and zinc in children seeking medical advice for attention-deficit/hyperactivity problems - an observational cohort study. *Lipids Health Dis.* 2010;9:105.

Notes

372   Rucklidge J, Taylor M, Whitehead K. Effect of micronutrients on behavior and mood in adults with ADHD: evidence from an 8-week open label trial with natural extension. *J Atten Disord.* 2011 Jan;15(1):79-91.

373   Rucklidge JJ, Frampton CM, Gorman B, Boggis A. Vitamin-mineral treatment of attention-deficit hyperactivity disorder in adults: double-blind randomised placebo-controlled trial. *Br J Psychiatry.* 2014;204:306-15.

374   Rucklidge JJ, Johnstone J, Kaplan BJ. Nutrient supplementation approaches in the treatment of ADHD. *Expert Rev Neurother.* 2009 Apr;9(4):461-76. doi: 10.1586/ern.09.7.

Chapter 12

375   Kingsley M. Effects of phosphatidylserine supplementation on exercising humans. *Sports Med.* 2006;36(8):657-69.

376   Kato-Kataoka A, Sakai M, Ebina R, Nonaka C, Asano T, Miyamori T. Soybean-derived phosphatidylserine improves memory function of the elderly Japanese subjects with memory complaints. *J Clin Biochem Nutr.* 2010 Nov;47(3):246-55.

377   Kato-Kataoka A, Sakai M, Ebina R, Nonaka C, Asano T, Miyamori T. Soybean-derived phosphatidylserine improves memory function of the elderly Japanese subjects with memory complaints. *J Clin Biochem Nutr.* 2010 Nov;47(3):246-55.

378   Doffek K, Chen X, Sugg SL, Shilyansky J. Phosphatidylserine inhibits NFκB and p38 MAPK activation in human monocyte derived dendritic cells. *Mol Immunol.* 2011 Sep;48(15-16):1771-7. doi:10.1016/j.molimm.2011.04.021.

379   Hoffmann PR, Kench JA, Vondracek A, et al. Interaction between phosphatidylserine and the phosphatidylserine receptor inhibits immune responses in vivo. *J Immunol.* 2005 Feb 1;174(3):1393-404.

380   GRAS Notices. GRN No. 279. Phosphatidylserine derived from fish. U.S. Food and Drug Administration website. http://www.accessdata.fda.gov/scripts/fdcc/index.cfm?set=GRASNotices&id=279. Updated October 30, 2015.

381   Kato-Kataoka A, Sakai M, Ebina R, Nonaka C, Asano T, Miyamori T. Soybean-derived phosphatidylserine improves memory function of the elderly Japanese subjects with memory complaints. *J Clin Biochem Nutr.* 2010 Nov;47(3):246-55.

382   Orologas AG, Buckman TD, Eiduson S. A comparison of platelet monoamine oxidase activity and phosphatidylserine content between chronic paranoid schizophrenics and normal controls. *Neurosci Lett.* 1986 Aug 4;68(3):293-8.

383   Gagné J, Giguère C, Tocco G, et al. Effect of phosphatidylserine on the binding properties of glutamate receptors in brain sections from adult and neonatal rats. *Brain Res.* 1996 Nov 18;740(1-2):337-45.

384   Gruber R, Sadeh A, Raviv A. Instability of sleep patterns in children with attention-deficit/hyperactivity disorder. *J Am Acad Child Adolesc Psychiatry.* 2000 Apr;39(4):495-501.

385   Brambilla F, Maggioni M, Panerai AE, Sacerdote P, Cenacchi T. Beta-endorphin concentration in peripheral blood mononuclear cells of elderly depressed patients--effects of phosphatidylserine therapy. *Neuropsychobiology.* 1996;34(1):18-21.

386   Kato-Kataoka A, Sakai M, Ebina R, Nonaka C, Asano T, Miyamori T. Soybean-derived phosphatidylserine improves memory function of the elderly Japanese subjects with memory complaints. *J Clin Biochem Nutr.* 2010 Nov;47(3):246-55.

387   Starks MA, Starks SL, Kingsley M, Purpura M, Jäger R. The effects of phosphatidylserine on endocrine response to moderate intensity exercise. *J Int Soc Sports Nutr.* 2008 Jul 28;5:11.

388   Hirayama S, Masuda Y, Rabeler R. Effect of phosphatidylserine administration on symptoms of attention-deficit/hyperactivity disorder in children. *Agro Food.* 2006;17(5):32-36.

389   Manor I, Magen A, Keidar D, et al. The effect of phosphatidylserine containing Omega3 fatty-acids on attention-deficit hyperactivity disorder symptoms in children: a double-blind placebo-controlled trial, followed by an open-label extension. *Eur Psychiatry.* 2012;27(5):335-42.

390   Manor I, Magen A, Keidar D, et al. Safety of phosphatidylserine containing omega3 fatty acids in ADHD children: a double-blind placebo-controlled trial followed by an open-label extension. *Eur Psychiatry.* 2013 Aug;28(6):386-91. doi: 10.1016/j.eurpsy.2012.11.001.

391   Hirayama S, Terasawa K, Rabeler R, et al. The effect of phosphatidylserine administration on memory and symptoms of attention-deficit hyperactivity disorder: a randomised, double-blind, placebo-controlled clinical trial. *J Hum Nutr Diet.* 2014;27(suppl 2):284-91.

392   Vaya Pharma website. http://www.vayapharma.com.

393   Hirayama S, Masuda Y, Rabeler R. Effect of phosphatidylserine administration on symptoms of attention-deficit/hyperactivity disorder in children. *Agro Food.* 2006;17(5):32-36.

394   GRAS Notices. GRN No. 279. Phosphatidylserine derived from fish. U.S. Food and Drug Administration website. http://www.accessdata.fda.gov/scripts/fdcc/index.cfm?set=GRASNotices&id=279. Updated October 30, 2015.

395   Vaya Pharma website. http://www.vayapharma.com.

396   Phosphatidylserine. Monograph. *Altern Med Rev.* 2008 Sep;13(3):245-7.

397   Phosphatidylserine. Monograph. *Altern Med Rev.* 2008 Sep;13(3):245-7.

398   Phosphatidylserine. Monograph. *Altern Med Rev.* 2008 Sep;13(3):245-7.

399   Tufekci O, Gunes D, Ozoğul C, et al. Evaluation of the effect of acetyl L-carnitine on experimental cisplatin nephrotoxicity. *Chemotherapy.* 2009;55(6):451-9. doi: 10.1159/000240020.

400   Liu J, Head E, Kuratsune H, Cotman CW, Ames BN. Comparison of the effects of L-carnitine and acetyl-L-carnitine on carnitine levels, ambulatory activity, and oxidative stress biomarkers in the brain of old rats. *Ann N Y Acad Sci.* 2004 Nov;1033:117-31.

401   Yasui F, Matsugo S, Ishibashi M, et al. Effects of chronic acetyl-L-carnitine treatment on brain lipid hydroperoxide level and passive avoidance learning in senescence-accelerated mice. *Neurosci Lett.* 2002 Dec 16;334(3):177-80.

402   Trebatická J, Kopasová S, Hradecná Z, et al. Treatment of ADHD with French maritime pine bark extract, Pycnogenol. *Eur Child Adolesc Psychiatry.* 2006 Sep;15(6):329-35.

403   Arduini A, Gorbunov N, Arrigoni-Martelli E, et al. Effects of L-carnitine and its acetate and propionate esters on the molecular dynamics of human erythrocyte membrane. *Biochim Biophys Acta.* 1993 Mar 14;1146(2):229-35.

Notes

404   Acetyl-L-carnitine. Monograph. *Altern Med Rev.* 2010 Apr;15(1):76-83.

405   Kobayashi S, Iwamoto M, Kon K, Waki H, Ando S, Tanaka Y. Acetyl-L-carnitine improves aged brain function. *Geriatr Gerontol Int.* 2010 Jul;10 Suppl 1:S99-106.

406   Taglialatela G, Navarra D, Cruciani R, Ramacci MT, Alemà GS, Angelucci L. Acetyl-L-carnitine treatment increases nerve growth factor levels and choline acetyltransferase activity in the central nervous system of aged rats. *Exp Gerontol.* 1994 Jan-Feb;29(1):55-66.

407   Smeland OB, Meisingset TW, Borges K, Sonnewald U. Chronic acetyl-L-carnitine alters brain energy metabolism and increases noradrenaline and serotonin content in healthy mice. *Neurochem Int.* 2012 Jul;61(1):100-7. doi: 10.1016/j.neuint.2012.04.008.

408   Harsing LG Jr, Sershen H, Toth E, Hashim A, Ramacci MT, Lajtha A. Acetyl-L-carnitine releases dopamine in rat corpus striatum: an in vivo microdialysis study. *Eur J Pharmacol.* 1992 Jul 21;218(1):117-21.

409   Sershen H, Harsing LG Jr, Banay-Schwartz M, Hashim A, Ramacci MT, Lajtha A. Effect of acetyl-L-carnitine on the dopaminergic system in aging brain. *J Neurosci Res.* 1991 Nov;30(3):555-9.

410   Tempesta E, Janiri L, Pirrongelli C. Stereospecific effects of acetylcarnitine on the spontaneous activity of brainstem neurones and their responses to acetylcholine and serotonin. *Neuropharmacology.* 1985 Jan;24(1):43-50.

411   Tolu P, Masi F, Leggio B, et al. Effects of long-term acetyl-L-carnitine administration in rats: I. increased dopamine output in mesocorticolimbic areas and protection toward acute stress exposure. *Neuropsychopharmacology.* 2002 Sep;27(3):410-20.

412   Tolu P, Masi F, Leggio B, et al. Effects of long-term acetyl-L-carnitine administration in rats: I. increased dopamine output in mesocorticolimbic areas and protection toward acute stress exposure. *Neuropsychopharmacology.* 2002 Sep;27(3):410-20.

413   Tolu P, Masi F, Leggio B, et al. Effects of long-term acetyl-L-carnitine administration in rats: I. increased dopamine output in mesocorticolimbic areas and protection toward acute stress exposure. *Neuropsychopharmacology.* 2002 Sep;27(3):410-20.

414   Tempesta E, Janiri L, Pirrongelli C. Stereospecific effects of acetylcarnitine on the spontaneous activity of brainstem neurones and their responses to acetylcholine and serotonin. *Neuropharmacology.* 1985 Jan;24(1):43-50.

415   Traina G, Federighi G, Brunelli M, Scuri R. Cytoprotective effect of acetyl-L-carnitine evidenced by analysis of gene expression in the rat brain. *Mol Neurobiol.* 2009 Apr;39(2):101-6.

416   Sharman EH, Vaziri ND, Ni Z, Sharman KG, Bondy SC. Reversal of biochemical and behavioral parameters of brain aging by melatonin and acetyl L-carnitine. *Brain Res.* 2002 Dec 13;957(2):223-30.

417   Tolu P, Masi F, Leggio B, et al. Effects of long-term acetyl-L-carnitine administration in rats: I. increased dopamine output in mesocorticolimbic areas and protection toward acute stress exposure. *Neuropsychopharmacology.* 2002 Sep;27(3):410-20.

418   Tempesta E, Casella L, Pirrongelli C, Janiri L, Calvani M, Ancona L. L-acetylcarnitine in depressed elderly subjects. A cross-over study vs placebo. *Drugs Exp Clin Res.* 1987;13(7):417-23.

235

419   Martinotti G, Andreoli S, Reina D, et al. Acetyl-l-Carnitine in the treatment of anhedonia, melancholic and negative symptoms in alcohol dependent subjects. *Prog Neuropsychopharmacol Biol Psychiatry.* 2011 Jun 1;35(4):953-8.

420   Bonavita E. Study of the efficacy and tolerability of L-acetylcarnitine therapy in the senile brain. *Int J Clin Pharmacol Ther Toxicol.* 1986 Sep;24(9):511-6.

421   Hao J, Shen W, Tian C, et al. Mitochondrial nutrients improve immune dysfunction in the type 2 diabetic Goto-Kakizaki rats. *J Cell Mol Med.* 2009 Apr;13(4):701-11. doi: 10.1111/j.1582-4934.2008.00342.x.

422   Vermeulen RC, Scholte HR. Exploratory open label, randomized study of acetyl- and propionylcarnitine in chronic fatigue syndrome. *Psychosom Med.* 2004 Mar-Apr;66(2):276-82.

423   Rossini M, Di Munno O, Valentini G, et al. Double-blind, multicenter trial comparing acetyl l-carnitine with placebo in the treatment of fibromyalgia patients. *Clin Exp Rheumatol.* 2007 Mar-Apr;25(2):182-8.

424   Beghi E, Pupillo E, Bonito V, et al. Randomized double-blind placebo-controlled trial of acetyl-L-carnitine for ALS. *Amyotroph Lateral Scler Frontotemporal Degener.* 2013 Sep;14(5-6):397-405. doi: 10.3109/21678421.2013.764568.

425   Van Oudheusden LJ, Scholte HR. Efficacy of carnitine in the treatment of children with attention-deficit hyperactivity disorder. *Prostaglandins Leukot Essent Fatty Acids.* 2002 Jul;67(1):33-8.

426   Taglialatela G, Navarra D, Cruciani R, Ramacci MT, Alemà GS, Angelucci L. Acetyl-L-carnitine treatment increases nerve growth factor levels and choline acetyltransferase activity in the central nervous system of aged rats. *Exp Gerontol.* 1994 Jan-Feb;29(1):55-66.

427   Arnold LE, Amato A, Bozzolo H, et al. Acetyl-L-carnitine (ALC) in attention-deficit/hyperactivity disorder: a multi-site, placebo-controlled pilot trial. *J Child Adolesc Psychopharmacol.* 2007 Dec;17(6):791-802.

428   Abbasi SH, Heidari S, Mohammadi MR, Tabrizi M, Ghaleiha A, Akhondzadeh S. Acetyl-L-carnitine as an adjunctive therapy in the treatment of attention-deficit/hyperactivity disorder in children and adolescents: a placebo-controlled trial. *Child Psychiatry Hum Dev.* 2011 Jun;42(3):367-75.

429   Torrioli MG, Vernacotola S, Peruzzi L, et al. A double-blind, parallel, multicenter comparison of L-acetylcarnitine with placebo on the attention deficit hyperactivity disorder in fragile X syndrome boys. *Am J Med Genet A.* 2008 Apr 1;146(7):803-12.

430   Sachan DS, Cha YS. Acetylcarnitine inhibits alcohol dehydrogenase. *Biochem Biophys Res Commun.* 1994 Sep 30;203(3):1496-501.

431   Caviglia D, Scarabelli L, Palmero S. Effects of carnitines on rat sertoli cell protein metabolism. *Horm Metab Res.* 2004 Apr;36(4):221-5.

432   Krsmanovic LZ, Virmani MA, Stojilkovic SS, Catt KJ. Stimulation of gonadotropin-releasing hormone secretion by acetyl-L-carnitine in hypothalamic neurons and GT1 neuronal cells. *Neurosci Lett.* 1994 Jan 3;165(1-2):33-6.

433   Krsmanović LZ, Virmani MA, Stojilković SS, Catt KJ. Actions of acetyl-L-carnitine on the hypothalamo-pituitary-gonadal system in female rats. *J Steroid Biochem Mol Biol.* 1992 Oct;43(4):351-8.

Notes

434   Genazzani AD, Lanzoni C, Ricchieri F, et al. Acetyl-L-carnitine (ALC) administration positively affects reproductive axis in hypogonadotropic women with functional hypothalamic amenorrhea. *J Endocrinol Invest.* 2011 Apr;34(4):287-91. doi: 10.3275/6997.

435   Sachan DS, Cha YS. Acetylcarnitine inhibits alcohol dehydrogenase. *Biochem Biophys Res Commun.* 1994 Sep 30;203(3):1496-501.

436   GRAS Notices. GRN No. 362. Levocarnitine. U.S. Food and Drug Administration website. http://www.accessdata.fda.gov/scripts/fdcc/index.cfm?set=GRASNotices&id=362. Updated October 30, 2015.

437   GRAS Notices. GRN No. 362. Levocarnitine. U.S. Food and Drug Administration website. http://www.accessdata.fda.gov/scripts/fdcc/index.cfm?set=GRASNotices&id=362. Updated October 30, 2015.

438   GRAS Notices. GRN No. 362. Levocarnitine. U.S. Food and Drug Administration website. http://www.accessdata.fda.gov/scripts/fdcc/index.cfm?set=GRASNotices&id=362. Updated October 30, 2015.

439   Evcimen H, Mania I, Mathews M, Basil B. Psychosis Precipitated by Acetyl-l-Carnitine in a Patient with Bipolar Disorder. *Prim Care Companion J Clin Psychiatry.* 2007; 9(1): 71-72.

440   Nicetile. TorrinoMedica website. http://www.torrinomedica.it/farmaci/ schedetecniche/Nicetile.asp#axzz40AhyY8LP. Updated January 12, 2007.

441   Dean O, Giorlando F, Berk M. N-acetylcysteine in psychiatry: current therapeutic evidence and potential mechanisms of action. *J Psychiatry Neurosci.* 2011 March; 36(2): 78-86.

442   Adair JC, Knoefel JE, Morgan N. Controlled trial of N-acetylcysteine for patients with probable Alzheimer's disease. *Neurology.* 2001 Oct 23;57(8):1515-7.

443   Adair JC, Knoefel JE, Morgan N. Controlled trial of N-acetylcysteine for patients with probable Alzheimer's disease. *Neurology.* 2001 Oct 23;57(8):1515-7.

444   Adair JC, Knoefel JE, Morgan N. Controlled trial of N-acetylcysteine for patients with probable Alzheimer's disease. *Neurology.* 2001 Oct 23;57(8):1515-7.

445   Magalhães PV, Dean OM, Bush AI, et al. N-acetylcysteine for major depressive episodes in bipolar disorder. *Rev Bras Psiquiatr.* 2011 Dec;33(4):374-8.

446   Lavoie S, Murray MM, Deppen P, et al. Glutathione precursor, N-acetyl-cysteine, improves mismatch negativity in schizophrenia patients. *Neuropsychopharmacology.* 2008 Aug;33(9):2187-99.

447   Adair JC, Knoefel JE, Morgan N. Controlled trial of N-acetylcysteine for patients with probable Alzheimer's disease. *Neurology.* 2001 Oct 23;57(8):1515-7.

448   Lafleur DL, Pittenger C, Kelmendi B, et al. N-acetylcysteine augmentation in serotonin reuptake inhibitor refractory obsessive-compulsive disorder. *Psychopharmacology (Berl).* 2006 Jan;184(2):254-6.

449   Grant JE, Odlaug BL, Kim SW. N-acetylcysteine, a glutamate modulator, in the treatment of trichotillomania: a double-blind, placebo-controlled study. *Arch Gen Psychiatry.* 2009 Jul;66(7):756-63.

450   Berk M, Jeavons S, Dean OM, et al. Nail-biting stuff? The effect of N-acetyl cysteine on nail-biting. *CNS Spectr.* 2009 Jul;14(7):357-60.

451   Grant JE, Kim SW, Odlaug BL. N-acetyl cysteine, a glutamate-modulating agent, in the treatment of pathological gambling: a pilot study. *Biol Psychiatry.* 2007 Sep 15;62(6):652-7.

452   Tayman C, Tonbul A, Kosus A, et al. N-acetylcysteine may prevent severe intestinal damage in necrotizing enterocolitis. *J Pediatr Surg.* 2012 Mar;47(3):540-50. doi: 10.1016/j.jpedsurg.2011.09.051.

453   Malins DC, Hellstrom KE, Anderson KM, Johnson PM, Vinson MA. Antioxidant-induced changes in oxidized DNA. *Proc Natl Acad Sci USA.* 2002 Apr 30;99(9):5937-41.

454   Chovanová Z, Muchová J, Sivonová M, et al. Effect of polyphenolic extract, Pycnogenol, on the level of 8-oxoguanine in children suffering from attention deficit/hyperactivity disorder. *Free Radic Res.* 2006 Sep;40(9):1003-10.

455   Martins MR, Reinke A, Petronilho FC, Gomes KM, Dal-Pizzol F, Quevedo J. Methylphenidate treatment induces oxidative stress in young rat brain. *Brain Res.* 2006 Mar 17;1078(1):189-97.

456   Bulut M, Selek S, Gergerlioglu HS, et al. Malondialdehyde levels in adult attention-deficit hyperactivity disorder. *J Psychiatry Neurosci.* 2007 Nov;32(6):435-8.

457   Bagh MB, Maiti AK, Jana S, Banerjee K, Roy A, Chakrabarti S. Quinone and oxyradical scavenging properties of N-acetylcysteine prevent dopamine mediated inhibition of Na+, K+-ATPase and mitochondrial electron transport chain activity in rat brain: implications in the neuroprotective therapy of Parkinson's disease. *Free Radic Res.* 2008 Jun;42(6):574-81. doi: 10.1080/10715760802158430.

458   Martins MR, Reinke A, Petronilho FC, Gomes KM, Dal-Pizzol F, Quevedo J. Methylphenidate treatment induces oxidative stress in young rat brain. *Brain Res.* 2006 Mar 17;1078(1):189-97.

459   Tocharus J, Khonthun C, Chongthammakun S, Govitrapong P. Melatonin attenuates methamphetamine-induced overexpression of pro-inflammatory cytokines in microglial cell lines. *J Pineal Res.* 2010 May;48(4):347-52.

460   El-Tawil OS, Abou-Hadeed AH, El-Bab MF, Shalaby AA. d-Amphetamine-induced cytotoxicity and oxidative stress in isolated rat hepatocytes. *Pathophysiology.* 2011 Sep;18(4):279-85.

461   Sae-Ung K, Uéda K, Govitrapong P, Phansuwan-Pujito P. Melatonin reduces the expression of alpha-synuclein in the dopamine containing neuronal regions of amphetamine-treated postnatal rats. *J Pineal Res.* 2012 Jan;52(1):128-37. doi: 10.1111/j.1600-079X.2011.00927.x.

462   Dvoráková M, Sivonová M, Trebatická J, et al. The effect of polyphenolic extract from pine bark, Pycnogenol on the level of glutathione in children suffering from attention deficit hyperactivity disorder (ADHD). *Redox Rep.* 2006;11(4):163-72.

463   Brawley A, Silverman B, Kearney S, et al. Allergic rhinitis in children with attention-deficit/hyperactivity disorder. *Ann Allergy Asthma Immunol.* 2004 Jun;92(6):663-7.

464   Jupp B, Caprioli D, Saigal N, et al. Dopaminergic and GABA-ergic markers of impulsivity in rats: evidence for anatomical localisation in ventral striatum and prefrontal cortex. *Eur J Neurosci.* 2013 Feb 1. doi: 10.1111/ejn.12146.

465   Carrey NJ, MacMaster FP, Gaudet L, Schmidt MH. Striatal creatine and glutamate/glutamine in attention-deficit/hyperactivity disorder. *J Child Adolesc Psychopharmacol.* 2007 Feb;17(1):11-7.

466   Carrey N, MacMaster FP, Sparkes SJ, Khan SC, Kusumakar V. Glutamatergic changes with treatment in attention deficit hyperactivity disorder: a preliminary case series. *J Child Adolesc Psychopharmacol.* 2002 Winter;12(4):331-6.

467   Kalivas PW. The glutamate homeostasis hypothesis of addiction. *Nat Rev Neurosci.* 2009 Aug;10(8):561-72. doi: 10.1038/nrn2515.

468   Schmaal L, Veltman DJ, Nederveen A, van den Brink W, Goudriaan AE. N-acetylcysteine normalizes glutamate levels in cocaine-dependent patients: a randomized crossover magnetic resonance spectroscopy study. *Neuropsychopharmacology.* 2012 Aug;37(9):2143-52. doi: 10.1038/npp.2012.66.

469   Garcia RJ, Francis L, Dawood M, Lai ZW, Faraone SV, Perl A. Attention deficit and hyperactivity disorder scores are elevated and respond to N-acetylcysteine treatment in patients with systemic lupus erythematosus. *Arthritis Rheum.* 2013 May;65(5):1313-8. doi: 10.1002/art.37893.

470   Hsu CC, Huang CN, Hung YC, Yin MC. Five cysteine-containing compounds have antioxidative activity in Balb/cA mice. *J Nutr.* 2004 Jan;134(1):149-52.

471   Demirkol O, Adams C, Ercal N. Biologically important thiols in various vegetables and fruits. *J Agric Food Chem.* 2004 Dec 29;52(26):8151-4.

472   Council for Responsible Nutrition: CRN List of Dietary Ingredients "Grandfathered" Under DHSEA. U.S. Food and Drug Administration website. http://www.fda.gov/ohrms/dockets/dockets/05p0305/05p-0305-cr00001-04-Council-For-Responsible-Nutrition-vol1.pdf. September 1998.

473   N-acetylcysteine. *Altern Med Rev.* 2000 Oct;5(5):467-71.

474   N-acetylcysteine. *Altern Med Rev.* 2000 Oct;5(5):467-71.

475   N-acetylcysteine. *Altern Med Rev.* 2000 Oct;5(5):467-71.

Chapter 13

476   Understanding Pine Bark Extract as an Alternative Treatment (Upbeat). Stanford School of Medicine, Program on Prevention Outcomes and Practices website. http://ppop.stanford.edu/documents/antioxidant-presentation.pdf. Updated July 15, 2008.

477   Pycnogenol. U.S. National Library of Medicine, MedlinePlus website. http://www.nlm.nih.gov/medlineplus/druginfo/natural/1019.html. Updated August 15, 2011.

478   Grimm T, Skrabala R, Chovanová Z, et al. Single and multiple dose pharmacokinetics of maritime pine bark extract (pycnogenol) after oral administration to healthy volunteers. *BMC Clin Pharmacol.* 2006 Aug 3;6:4.

479   Ryan J, Croft K, Mori T, et al. An examination of the effects of the antioxidant Pycnogenol on cognitive performance, serum lipid profile, endocrinological and oxidative stress biomarkers in an elderly population. *J Psychopharmacol.* 2008 Jul;22(5):553-62.

480   Nelson AB, Lau BH, Ide N, Rong Y. Pycnogenol inhibits macrophage oxidative burst, lipoprotein oxidation, and hydroxyl radical-induced DNA damage. *Drug Dev Ind Pharm.* 1998 Feb;24(2):139-44.

481   Chovanová Z, Muchová J, Sivonová M, et al. Effect of polyphenolic extract, Pycnogenol, on the level of 8-oxoguanine in children suffering from attention deficit/hyperactivity disorder. *Free Radic Res.* 2006 Sep;40(9):1003-10.

482   Choi YH, Yan GH. Pycnogenol inhibits immunoglobulin E-mediated allergic response in mast cells. *Phytother Res.* 2009 Dec;23(12):1691-5.

483   Sivonová M, Waczulíková I, Kilanczyk E, et al. The effect of Pycnogenol on the erythrocyte membrane fluidity. *Gen Physiol Biophys.* 2004 Mar;23(1):39-51.

484   Tenenbaum S, Paull JC, Sparrow EP, Dodd DK, Green L. An experimental comparison of Pycnogenol and methylphenidate in adults with Attention-Deficit/Hyperactivity Disorder (ADHD). *J Atten Disord.* 2002 Sep;6(2):49-60.

485   Trebatická J, Kopasová S, Hradecná Z, et al. Treatment of ADHD with French maritime pine bark extract, Pycnogenol. *Eur Child Adolesc Psychiatry.* 2006 Sep;15(6):329-35.

486   Dvoráková M, Sivonová M, Trebatická J, et al. The effect of polyphenolic extract from pine bark, Pycnogenol on the level of glutathione in children suffering from attention deficit hyperactivity disorder (ADHD). *Redox Rep.* 2006;11(4):163-72.

487   Chovanová Z, Muchová J, Sivonová M, et al. Effect of polyphenolic extract, Pycnogenol, on the level of 8-oxoguanine in children suffering from attention deficit/hyperactivity disorder. *Free Radic Res.* 2006 Sep;40(9):1003-10.

488   Chovanová Z, Muchová J, Sivonová M, et al. Effect of polyphenolic extract, Pycnogenol, on the level of 8-oxoguanine in children suffering from attention deficit/hyperactivity disorder. *Free Radic Res.* 2006 Sep;40(9):1003-10.

489   Module 19. Botanicals Generally Recognized as Safe. United States Department of Agriculture, Agriculture Research Service website. https://www.fda.gov/downloads/Food/IngredientsPackagingLabeling/GRAS/NoticeInventory/ucm261591.pdf. Updated April 30, 2013.

490   Stanford School of Medicine, Program on Prevention Outcomes and Practices website. Pine Bark Research Study / Stanford Antioxidant Natural Supplement Study. http://ppop.stanford.edu/pinebark.html. Updated August 31, 2009.

491   Tenenbaum S, Paull JC, Sparrow EP, Dodd DK, Green L. An experimental comparison of Pycnogenol and methylphenidate in adults with Attention-Deficit/Hyperactivity Disorder (ADHD). *J Atten Disord.* 2002 Sep;6(2):49-60.

492   Stanford School of Medicine, Program on Prevention Outcomes and Practices website. Pine Bark Research Study / Stanford Antioxidant Natural Supplement Study. http://ppop.stanford.edu/pinebark.html. Updated August 31, 2009.

493   Stanford School of Medicine, Program on Prevention Outcomes and Practices website. Pine Bark Research Study / Stanford Antioxidant Natural Supplement Study. http://ppop.stanford.edu/pinebark.html. Updated August 31, 2009.

494   Trebatická J, Kopasová S, Hradecná Z, et al. Treatment of ADHD with French maritime pine bark extract, Pycnogenol. *Eur Child Adolesc Psychiatry.* 2006 Sep;15(6):329-35.

495   Tenenbaum S, Paull JC, Sparrow EP, Dodd DK, Green L. An experimental comparison of Pycnogenol and methylphenidate in adults with Attention-Deficit/Hyperactivity Disorder (ADHD). *J Atten Disord.* 2002 Sep;6(2):49-60.

496   Tenenbaum S, Paull JC, Sparrow EP, Dodd DK, Green L. An experimental comparison of Pycnogenol and methylphenidate in adults with Attention-Deficit/Hyperactivity Disorder (ADHD). *J Atten Disord.* 2002 Sep;6(2):49-60.

497   Smith JV, Luo Y. Studies on molecular mechanisms of Ginkgo biloba extract. *Appl Microbiol Biotechnol.* 2004 May;64(4):465-72.

Notes

498   Ude C, Schubert-Zsilavecz M, Wurglics M. Ginkgo biloba extracts: a review of the pharmacokinetics of the active ingredients. *Clin Pharmacokinet.* 2013;52(9):727-49.

499   Chan PC, Xia Q, Fu PP. Ginkgo biloba leave extract: biological, medicinal, and toxicological effects. *J Environ Sci Health C Environ Carcinog Ecotoxicol Rev.* 2007 Jul-Sep;25(3):211-44.

500   Rojas P, Serrano-García N, Medina-Campos ON, Pedraza-Chaverri J, Ogren SO, Rojas C. Antidepressant-like effect of a Ginkgo biloba extract (EGb761) in the mouse forced swimming test: role of oxidative stress. *Neurochem Int.* 2011 Oct;59(5):628-36. doi: 10.1016/j.neuint.2011.05.007.

501   Drieu K, Vranckx R, Benassayad C, et al. Effect of the extract of Ginkgo biloba (EGb 761) on the circulating and cellular profiles of polyunsaturated fatty acids: correlation with the anti-oxidant properties of the extract. *Prostaglandins Leukot Essent Fatty Acids.* 2000 Nov;63(5):293-300.

502   Drieu K, Vranckx R, Benassayad C, et al. Effect of the extract of Ginkgo biloba (EGb 761) on the circulating and cellular profiles of polyunsaturated fatty acids: correlation with the anti-oxidant properties of the extract. *Prostaglandins Leukot Essent Fatty Acids.* 2000 Nov;63(5):293-300.

503   Rojas P, Serrano-García N, Medina-Campos ON, Pedraza-Chaverri J, Ogren SO, Rojas C. Antidepressant-like effect of a Ginkgo biloba extract (EGb761) in the mouse forced swimming test: role of oxidative stress. *Neurochem Int.* 2011 Oct;59(5):628-36. doi: 10.1016/j.neuint.2011.05.007.

504   Smith JV, Luo Y. Studies on molecular mechanisms of Ginkgo biloba extract. *Appl Microbiol Biotechnol.* 2004 May;64(4):465-72.

505   Eckert A, Keil U, Kressmann S, et al. Effects of EGb 761 Ginkgo biloba extract on mitochondrial function and oxidative stress. *Pharmacopsychiatry.* 2003 Jun;36 Suppl 1:S15-23.

506   Rojas P, Serrano-García N, Medina-Campos ON, Pedraza-Chaverri J, Ogren SO, Rojas C. Antidepressant-like effect of a Ginkgo biloba extract (EGb761) in the mouse forced swimming test: role of oxidative stress. *Neurochem Int.* 2011 Oct;59(5):628-36. doi: 10.1016/j.neuint.2011.05.007.

507   Leistner E, Drewke C. Ginkgo biloba and ginkgotoxin. *J Nat Prod.* 2010 Jan;73(1):86-92. doi: 10.1021/np9005019.

508   Drieu K, Vranckx R, Benassayad C, et al. Effect of the extract of Ginkgo biloba (EGb 761) on the circulating and cellular profiles of polyunsaturated fatty acids: correlation with the anti-oxidant properties of the extract. *Prostaglandins Leukot Essent Fatty Acids.* 2000 Nov;63(5):293-300.

509   Rojas P, Serrano-García N, Medina-Campos ON, Pedraza-Chaverri J, Ogren SO, Rojas C. Antidepressant-like effect of a Ginkgo biloba extract (EGb761) in the mouse forced swimming test: role of oxidative stress. *Neurochem Int.* 2011 Oct;59(5):628-36. doi: 10.1016/j.neuint.2011.05.007.

510   Thanoon IA, Abdul-Jabbar HA, Taha DA. Oxidative Stress and C-Reactive Protein in Patients with Cerebrovascular Accident (Ischaemic Stroke): The role of Ginkgo biloba extract. *Sultan Qaboos Univ Med J.* 2012 May;12(2):197-205.

511   Matsushima H, Morimoto K. The modulation of immunological activities in human NK cells by extracts of ginkgo. *Environ Health Prev Med*. 2009 Nov;14(6):361-5. doi: 10.1007/s12199-009-0102-0.

512   Puebla-Pérez AM, Lozoya X, Villaseñor-García MM. Effect of Ginkgo biloba extract, EGb 761, on the cellular immune response in a hypothalamic-pituitary-adrenal axis activation model in the rat. *Int Immunopharmacol*. 2003 Jan;3(1):75-80.

513   Smith JV, Luo Y. Studies on molecular mechanisms of Ginkgo biloba extract. *Appl Microbiol Biotechnol*. 2004 May;64(4):465-72.

514   Qin XS, Jin KH, Ding BK, Xie SF, Ma H. Effects of extract of Ginkgo biloba with venlafaxine on brain injury in a rat model of depression. *Chin Med J (Engl)*. 2005 Mar 5;118(5):391-7.

515   Chandrasekaran K, Mehrabian Z, Spinnewyn B, Chinopoulos C, Drieu K, Fiskum G. Neuroprotective effects of bilobalide, a component of Ginkgo biloba extract (EGb 761) in global brain ischemia and in excitotoxicity-induced neuronal death. *Pharmacopsychiatry*. 2003 Jun;36 Suppl 1:S89-94.

516   Kiewert C, Kumar V, Hildmann O, Hartmann J, Hillert M, Klein J. Role of glycine receptors and glycine release for the neuroprotective activity of bilobalide. *Brain Res*. 2008 Mar 27;1201:143-50. doi: 10.1016/j.brainres.2008.01.052.

517   Rojas P, Serrano-García N, Medina-Campos ON, Pedraza-Chaverri J, Ogren SO, Rojas C. Antidepressant-like effect of a Ginkgo biloba extract (EGb761) in the mouse forced swimming test: role of oxidative stress. *Neurochem Int*. 2011 Oct;59(5):628-36. doi: 10.1016/j.neuint.2011.05.007.

518   Rojas P, Serrano-García N, Medina-Campos ON, Pedraza-Chaverri J, Ogren SO, Rojas C. Antidepressant-like effect of a Ginkgo biloba extract (EGb761) in the mouse forced swimming test: role of oxidative stress. *Neurochem Int*. 2011 Oct;59(5):628-36. doi: 10.1016/j.neuint.2011.05.007.

519   Hemmeter U, Annen B, Bischof R, et al. Polysomnographic effects of adjuvant ginkgo biloba therapy in patients with major depression medicated with trimipramine. *Pharmacopsychiatry*. 2001 Mar;34(2):50-9.

520   Jezova D, Duncko R, Lassanova M, Kriska M, Moncek F. Reduction of rise in blood pressure and cortisol release during stress by Ginkgo biloba extract (EGb 761) in healthy volunteers. *J Physiol Pharmacol*. 2002 Sep;53(3):337-48.

521   Walesiuk A, Braszko JJ. Gingkoselect alleviates chronic corticosterone-induced spatial memory deficits in rats. *Fitoterapia*. 2010 Jan;81(1):25-9. doi: 10.1016/j.fitote.2009.06.020.

522   Bolaños-Jiménez F, Manhães de Castro R, Sarhan H, Prudhomme N, Drieu K, Fillion G. Stress-induced 5-HT1A receptor desensitization: protective effects of Ginkgo biloba extract (EGb 761). *Fundam Clin Pharmacol*. 1995;9(2):169-74.

523   Rojas P, Serrano-García N, Medina-Campos ON, Pedraza-Chaverri J, Ogren SO, Rojas C. Antidepressant-like effect of a Ginkgo biloba extract (EGb761) in the mouse forced swimming test: role of oxidative stress. *Neurochem Int*. 2011 Oct;59(5):628-36. doi: 10.1016/j.neuint.2011.05.007.

524   Kehr J, Yoshitake S, Ijiri S, Koch E, Nöldner M, Yoshitake T. Ginkgo biloba leaf extract (EGb 761®) and its specific acylated flavonol constituents increase dopamine and acetyl-

choline levels in the rat medial prefrontal cortex: possible implications for the cognitive enhancing properties of EGb 761°. *Int Psychogeriatr.* 2012 Aug;24 Suppl 1:S25-34. doi: 10.1017/S1041610212000567.

525   Yoshitake T, Yoshitake S, Kehr J. The Ginkgo biloba extract EGb 761(R) and its main constituent flavonoids and ginkgolides increase extracellular dopamine levels in the rat prefrontal cortex. *Br J Pharmacol.* 2010 Feb 1;159(3):659-68. doi: 10.1111/j.1476-5381.2009.00580.x.

526   Fehske CJ, Leuner K, Müller WE. Ginkgo biloba extract (EGb761) influences monoaminergic neurotransmission via inhibition of NE uptake, but not MAO activity after chronic treatment. *Pharmacol Res.* 2009 Jul;60(1):68-73. doi: 10.1016/j.phrs.2009.02.012.

527   Huguet F, Drieu K, Piriou A. Decreased cerebral 5-HT1A receptors during ageing: reversal by Ginkgo biloba extract (EGb 761). *J Pharm Pharmacol.* 1994 Apr;46(4):316-8.

528   Sasaki K, Hatta S, Wada K, Ohshika H, Haga M. Bilobalide prevents reduction of gamma-aminobutyric acid levels and glutamic acid decarboxylase activity induced by 4-O-methylpyridoxine in mouse hippocampus. *Life Sci.* 2000 Jun 30;67(6):709-15.

529   Sasaki K, Hatta S, Wada K, Itoh M, Yoshimura T, Haga M. Effects of chronic administration of bilobalide on amino acid levels in mouse brain. *Cell Mol Biol (Noisy-le-grand).* 2002 Sep;48(6):681-4.

530   Ivic L, Sands TT, Fishkin N, Nakanishi K, Kriegstein AR, Strømgaard K. Terpene trilactones from Ginkgo biloba are antagonists of cortical glycine and GABA(A) receptors. *J Biol Chem.* 2003 Dec 5;278(49):49279-85.

531   Xiao ZY, Sun CK, Xiao XW, et al. Effects of Ginkgo biloba extract against excitotoxicity induced by NMDA receptors and mechanism thereof. *Zhonghua Yi Xue Za Zhi.* 2006 Sep 19;86(35):2479-84.

532   Kiewert C, Kumar V, Hildmann O, et al. Role of GABAergic antagonism in the neuroprotective effects of bilobalide. *Brain Res.* 2007 Jan 12;1128(1):70-8.

533   Rojas P, Serrano-García N, Medina-Campos ON, Pedraza-Chaverri J, Ogren SO, Rojas C. Antidepressant-like effect of a Ginkgo biloba extract (EGb761) in the mouse forced swimming test: role of oxidative stress. *Neurochem Int.* 2011 Oct;59(5):628-36. doi: 10.1016/j.neuint.2011.05.007.

534   Walesiuk A, Braszko JJ. Gingkoselect alleviates chronic corticosterone-induced spatial memory deficits in rats. *Fitoterapia.* 2010 Jan;81(1):25-9. doi: 10.1016/j.fitote.2009.06.020.

535   Stoll S, Scheuer K, Pohl O, Müller WE. Ginkgo biloba extract (EGb 761) independently improves changes in passive avoidance learning and brain membrane fluidity in the aging mouse. *Pharmacopsychiatry.* 1996 Jul;29(4):144-9.

536   Carlson JJ, Farquhar JW, DiNucci E, et al. Safety and efficacy of a ginkgo biloba-containing dietary supplement on cognitive function, quality of life, and platelet function in healthy, cognitively intact older adults. *J Am Diet Assoc.* 2007 Mar;107(3):422-32.

537   Horsch S, Walther C. Ginkgo biloba special extract EGb 761 in the treatment of peripheral arterial occlusive disease (PAOD)--a review based on randomized, controlled studies. *Int J Clin Pharmacol Ther.* 2004 Feb;42(2):63-72.

538   Rojas P, Serrano-García N, Medina-Campos ON, Pedraza-Chaverri J, Ogren SO, Rojas C. Antidepressant-like effect of a Ginkgo biloba extract (EGb761) in the mouse forced swimming test: role of oxidative stress. *Neurochem Int.* 2011 Oct;59(5):628-36. doi: 10.1016/j.neuint.2011.05.007.

539   Amin A, Abraham C, Hamza AA, et al. A standardized extract of Ginkgo biloba neutralizes cisplatin-mediated reproductive toxicity in rats. *J Biomed Biotechnol.* 2012;2012:362049. doi: 10.1155/2012/362049.

540   Zhang L, Mao W, Guo X, et al. Ginkgo biloba Extract for Patients with Early Diabetic Nephropathy: A Systematic Review. *Evid Based Complement Alternat Med.* 2013;2013:689142. doi: 10.1155/2013/689142.

541   Hamann KF. Special ginkgo extract in cases of vertigo: a systematic review of randomised, double-blind, placebo controlled clinical examinations. *HNO.* 2007 Apr;55(4):258-63.

542   Tang Y, Xu Y, Xiong S, et al. The effect of Ginkgo Biloba extract on the expression of PKCalpha in the inflammatory cells and the level of IL-5 in induced sputum of asthmatic patients. *J Huazhong Univ Sci Technolog Med Sci.* 2007 Aug;27(4):375-80.

543   Ozgoli G, Selselei EA, Mojab F, Majd HA. A randomized, placebo-controlled trial of Ginkgo biloba L. in treatment of premenstrual syndrome. *J Altern Complement Med.* 2009 Aug;15(8):845-51. doi: 10.1089/acm.2008.0493.

544   Meston CM, Rellini AH, Telch MJ. Short- and long-term effects of Ginkgo biloba extract on sexual dysfunction in women. *Arch Sex Behav.* 2008 Aug;37(4):530-47. doi: 10.1007/s10508-008-9316-2.

545   Cohen AJ, Bartlik B. Ginkgo biloba for antidepressant-induced sexual dysfunction. *J Sex Marital Ther.* 1998 Apr-Jun;24(2):139-43.

546   Fehske CJ, Leuner K, Müller WE. Ginkgo biloba extract (EGb761) influences monoaminergic neurotransmission via inhibition of NE uptake, but not MAO activity after chronic treatment. *Pharmacol Res.* 2009 Jul;60(1):68-73. doi: 10.1016/j.phrs.2009.02.012.

547   Woelk H, Arnoldt KH, Kieser M, Hoerr R. Ginkgo biloba special extract EGb 761 in generalized anxiety disorder and adjustment disorder with anxious mood: a randomized, double-blind, placebo-controlled trial. *J Psychiatr Res.* 2007 Sep;41(6):472-80.

548   Singh V, Singh SP, Chan K. Review and meta-analysis of usage of ginkgo as an adjunct therapy in chronic schizophrenia. *Int J Neuropsychopharmacol.* 2010 Mar;13(2):257-71. doi: 10.1017/S1461145709990654.

549   Weinmann S, Roll S, Schwarzbach C, Vauth C, Willich SN. Effects of Ginkgo biloba in dementia: systematic review and meta-analysis. *BMC Geriatr.* 2010 Mar 17;10:14. doi: 10.1186/1471-2318-10-14.

550   Vellas B, Coley N, Ousset PJ, et al. Long-term use of standardised Ginkgo biloba extract for the prevention of Alzheimer's disease (GuidAge): a randomised placebo-controlled trial. *Lancet Neurol.* 2012 Oct;11(10):851-9. doi: 10.1016/S1474-4422(12)70206-5.

551   Ginkgo. National Institute of Environmental Health Sciences NIH-HHS website. http://www.niehs.nih.gov/health/topics/agents/ginkgo/index.cfm. Updated February 4, 2016.

Notes

552   Kaschel R. Ginkgo biloba: specificity of neuropsychological improvement--a selective review in search of differential effects. *Hum Psychopharmacol.* 2009 Jul;24(5):345-70. doi: 10.1002/hup.1037.

553   Ozgoli G, Selselei EA, Mojab F, Majd HA. A randomized, placebo-controlled trial of Ginkgo biloba L. in treatment of premenstrual syndrome. *J Altern Complement Med.* 2009 Aug;15(8):845-51. doi: 10.1089/acm.2008.0493.

554   Cieza A, Maier P, Pöppel E. Effects of Ginkgo biloba on mental functioning in healthy volunteers. *Arch Med Res.* 2003 Sep-Oct;34(5):373-81.

555   Drieu K, Vranckx R, Benassayad C, et al. Effect of the extract of Ginkgo biloba (EGb 761) on the circulating and cellular profiles of polyunsaturated fatty acids: correlation with the anti-oxidant properties of the extract. *Prostaglandins Leukot Essent Fatty Acids.* 2000 Nov;63(5):293-300.

556   Eckert A, Keil U, Kressmann S, et al. Effects of EGb 761 Ginkgo biloba extract on mitochondrial function and oxidative stress. *Pharmacopsychiatry.* 2003 Jun;36 Suppl 1:S15-23.

557   National Toxicology Program. Toxicology and Carcinogenesis Studies of Ginkgo biloba Extract (CAS No. 90045-36-6) in F344/N Rats and B6C3F1/N Mice (Gavage studies). *Natl Toxicol Program Tech Rep Ser.* 2013 Mar;(578):1-184.

558   Eckert A, Keil U, Kressmann S, et al. Effects of EGb 761 Ginkgo biloba extract on mitochondrial function and oxidative stress. *Pharmacopsychiatry.* 2003 Jun;36 Suppl 1:S15-23.

559   Kellermann AJ, Kloft C. Is there a risk of bleeding associated with standardized Ginkgo biloba extract therapy? A systematic review and metaanalysis. *Pharmacotherapy.* 2011 May;31(5):490-502. doi: 10.1592/phco.31.5.490.

560   Rojas P, Serrano-García N, Medina-Campos ON, Pedraza-Chaverri J, Ogren SO, Rojas C. Antidepressant-like effect of a Ginkgo biloba extract (EGb761) in the mouse forced swimming test: role of oxidative stress. *Neurochem Int.* 2011 Oct;59(5):628-36. doi: 10.1016/j.neuint.2011.05.007.

561   Drieu K, Vranckx R, Benassayad C, et al. Effect of the extract of Ginkgo biloba (EGb 761) on the circulating and cellular profiles of polyunsaturated fatty acids: correlation with the anti-oxidant properties of the extract. *Prostaglandins Leukot Essent Fatty Acids.* 2000 Nov;63(5):293-300.

562   Dugoua JJ, Mills E, Perri D, Koren G. Safety and efficacy of ginkgo (Ginkgo biloba) during pregnancy and lactation. *Can J Clin Pharmacol.* 2006 Fall;13(3):e277-84.

563   Salehi B, Imani R, Mohammadi MR, et al. Ginkgo biloba for attention-deficit/hyperactivity disorder in children and adolescents: a double blind, randomized controlled trial. *Prog Neuropsychopharmacol Biol Psychiatry.* 2010 Feb 1;34(1):76-80. doi: 10.1016/j.pnpbp.2009.09.026.

564   Tada Y, Kagota S, Kubota Y, et al. Long-term feeding of Ginkgo biloba extract impairs peripheral circulation and hepatic function in aged spontaneously hypertensive rats. *Biol Pharm Bull.* 2008 Jan;31(1):68-72.

565   Fontana L, Souza AS, Del Bel EA, Oliveira RM. Ginkgo biloba leaf extract (EGb 761) enhances catalepsy induced by haloperidol and L-nitroarginine in mice. *Braz J Med Biol Res.* 2005 Nov;38(11):1649-54.

566   Cianfrocca C, Pelliccia F, Auriti A, Santini M. Ginkgo biloba-induced frequent ventricular arrhythmia. *Ital Heart J.* 2002 Nov;3(11):689-91.

567   Yeh KY, Pu HF, Kaphle K, et al. Ginkgo biloba extract enhances male copulatory behavior and reduces serum prolactin levels in rats. *Horm Behav.* 2008 Jan;53(1):225-31.

568   Yeh KY, Wu CH, Tai MY, Tsai YF. Ginkgo biloba extract enhances noncontact erection in rats: the role of dopamine in the paraventricular nucleus and the mesolimbic system. *Neuroscience.* 2011 Aug 25;189:199-206. doi: 10.1016/j.neuroscience.2011.05.025.

569   Salehi B, Imani R, Mohammadi MR, et al. Ginkgo biloba for attention-deficit/hyperactivity disorder in children and adolescents: a double blind, randomized controlled trial. *Prog Neuropsychopharmacol Biol Psychiatry.* 2010 Feb 1;34(1):76-80. doi: 10.1016/j.pnpbp.2009.09.026.

570   Salehi B, Imani R, Mohammadi MR, et al. Ginkgo biloba for attention-deficit/hyperactivity disorder in children and adolescents: a double blind, randomized controlled trial. *Prog Neuropsychopharmacol Biol Psychiatry.* 2010 Feb 1;34(1):76-80. doi: 10.1016/j.pnpbp.2009.09.026.

571   Salehi B, Imani R, Mohammadi MR, et al. Ginkgo biloba for attention-deficit/hyperactivity disorder in children and adolescents: a double blind, randomized controlled trial. *Prog Neuropsychopharmacol Biol Psychiatry.* 2010 Feb 1;34(1):76-80. doi: 10.1016/j.pnpbp.2009.09.026.

572   Wu XY, Wang WY, Wang RR, Xie L, Fang ZX, Chen GR. Ginkgo biloba extract enhances testosterone synthesis of Leydig cells in type 2 diabetic rats. *Zhonghua Nan Ke Xue.* 2008 Apr;14(4):371-6.

573   Markowitz JS, DeVane CL, Lewis JG, Chavin KD, Wang JS, Donovan JL. Effect of Ginkgo biloba extract on plasma steroid concentrations in healthy volunteers: a pilot study. *Pharmacotherapy.* 2005 Oct;25(10):1337-40.

574   Niederhofer H. Ginkgo biloba treating patients with attention-deficit disorder. *Phytother Res.* 2010 Jan;24(1):26-7. doi: 10.1002/ptr.2854.

575   Salehi B, Imani R, Mohammadi MR, et al. Ginkgo biloba for attention-deficit/hyperactivity disorder in children and adolescents: a double blind, randomized controlled trial. *Prog Neuropsychopharmacol Biol Psychiatry.* 2010 Feb 1;34(1):76-80. doi: 10.1016/j.pnpbp.2009.09.026.

576   Katz M, Levine AA, Kol-Degani H, Kav-Venaki L. A compound herbal preparation (CHP) in the treatment of children with ADHD: a randomized controlled trial. *J Atten Disord.* 2010 Nov;14(3):281-91. doi: 10.1177/1087054709356388.

577   Monograph. Peony. *Altern Med Rev.* 2001 Oct;6(5):495-9.

578   Sun R, Wang K, Wu D, Li X, Ou Y. Protective effect of paeoniflorin against glutamate-induced neurotoxicity in PC12 cells via Bcl-2/Bax signal pathway. *Folia Neuropathol.* 2012;50(3):270-6.

579   Qiu FM, Zhong XM, Mao QQ, Huang Z. Antidepressant-like effects of paeoniflorin on the behavioural, biochemical, and neurochemical patterns of rats exposed to chronic unpredictable stress. *Neurosci Lett.* 2013 Apr 29;541:209-13. doi: 10.1016/j.neulet.2013.02.029.

Notes

580   Yang Q, Yang L, Xiong A, Lu L, Wang R, Wang Z. Metabolomics study of anti-in-flammatory action of Radix Paeoniae Rubra and Radix Paeoniae Alba by ultraperfor-mance liquid chromatography-mass spectrometry. *Zhongguo Zhong Yao Za Zhi.* 2011 Mar;36(6):694-7.

581   Zhu Y, Dang S, Hua Z. Advanced achievements about neuroprotective mecha-nisms of paeoniflorin. *Zhongguo Zhong Yao Za Zhi.* 2010 Jun;35(11):1490-3.

582   Huang KS, Lin JG, Lee HC, et al. Paeoniae alba Radix Promotes Peripheral Nerve Regeneration. *Evid Based Complement Alternat Med.* 2011;2011:109809. doi: 10.1093/ecam/nep115.

583   Qiu F, Zhong X, Mao Q, Huang Z. The antidepressant-like effects of paeoniflorin in mouse models. *Exp Ther Med.* 2013 Apr;5(4):1113-1116.

584   Qiu FM, Zhong XM, Mao QQ, Huang Z. Antidepressant-like effects of paeoniflorin on the behavioural, biochemical, and neurochemical patterns of rats exposed to chronic unpredictable stress. *Neurosci Lett.* 2013 Apr 29;541:209-13. doi: 10.1016/j.neulet.2013.02.029.

585   Qiu FM, Zhong XM, Mao QQ, Huang Z. Antidepressant-like effects of paeoniflorin on the behavioural, biochemical, and neurochemical patterns of rats exposed to chronic unpredictable stress. *Neurosci Lett.* 2013 Apr 29;541:209-13. doi: 10.1016/j.neulet.2013.02.029.

586   Liu TP, Liu M, Tsai CC, Lai TY, Hsu FL, Cheng JT. Stimulatory effect of paeoniflorin on the release of noradrenaline from ileal synaptosomes of guinea-pig in-vitro. *J Pharm Pharmacol.* 2002 May;54(5):681-8.

587   Qiu FM, Zhong XM, Mao QQ, Huang Z. Antidepressant-like effects of paeoniflorin on the behavioural, biochemical, and neurochemical patterns of rats exposed to chronic unpredictable stress. *Neurosci Lett.* 2013 Apr 29;541:209-13. doi: 10.1016/j.neulet.2013.02.029.

588   Qiu FM, Zhong XM, Mao QQ, Huang Z. Antidepressant-like effects of paeoniflo-rin on the behavioural, biochemical, and neurochemical patterns of rats exposed to chronic unpredictable stress. *Neurosci Lett.* 2013 Apr 29;541:209-13. doi: 10.1016/j.neulet.2013.02.029.

589   U.S. Food and Drug Administration website. https://www.accessdata.fda.gov/scripts/fdcc/?set=GRASNotices&sort=GRN_No&order=DESC&startrow=1&type=ba-sic&search=peony. March 31, 2016.

590   Peony. WebMD website. http://www.webmd.com/vitamins-supplements/ingredi-entmono-32-PEONY.aspx?activeIngredientId=32&activeIngredientName=PEONY. Updated 2009.

591   Qiu FM, Zhong XM, Mao QQ, Huang Z. Antidepressant-like effects of paeoniflo-rin on the behavioural, biochemical, and neurochemical patterns of rats exposed to chronic unpredictable stress. *Neurosci Lett.* 2013 Apr 29;541:209-13. doi: 10.1016/j.neulet.2013.02.029.

592   Qiu FM, Zhong XM, Mao QQ, Huang Z. Antidepressant-like effects of paeoniflo-rin on the behavioural, biochemical, and neurochemical patterns of rats exposed to chronic unpredictable stress. *Neurosci Lett.* 2013 Apr 29;541:209-13. doi: 10.1016/j.neulet.2013.02.029.

593   Qiu FM, Zhong XM, Mao QQ, Huang Z. Antidepressant-like effects of paeoniflo-rin on the behavioural, biochemical, and neurochemical patterns of rats exposed to chronic unpredictable stress. *Neurosci Lett.* 2013 Apr 29;541:209-13. doi: 10.1016/j.neulet.2013.02.029.

594   Qiu FM, Zhong XM, Mao QQ, Huang Z. Antidepressant-like effects of paeoniflo-rin on the behavioural, biochemical, and neurochemical patterns of rats exposed to chronic unpredictable stress. *Neurosci Lett.* 2013 Apr 29;541:209-13. doi: 10.1016/j.neulet.2013.02.029.

595   Qiu FM, Zhong XM, Mao QQ, Huang Z. Antidepressant-like effects of paeoniflo-rin on the behavioural, biochemical, and neurochemical patterns of rats exposed to chronic unpredictable stress. *Neurosci Lett.* 2013 Apr 29;541:209-13. doi: 10.1016/j.neulet.2013.02.029.

596   Peony. WebMD website. http://www.webmd.com/vitamins-supplements/ingredientmono-32-PEONY.aspx?activeIngredientId=32&activeIngredientName=PEONY. Updated 2009.

597   Takeuchi T. Effect of shakuyaku-kanzo-to, shakuyaku, kanzo, paeoniflorin, glycyr-rhetinic acid and glycyrrhizin on ovarian function in rats. *Nihon Naibunpi Gakkai Zasshi.* 1988 Nov 20;64(11):1124-39.

598   Monograph. Withania somnifera. *Altern Med Rev.* 2004 Jun;9(2):211-4.

599   Mishra LC, Singh BB, Dagenais S. Scientific basis for the therapeutic use of Witha-nia somnifera (ashwagandha): a review. *Altern Med Rev.* 2000 Aug;5(4):334-46.

600   Ahmad MK, Mahdi AA, Shukla KK, et al. Withania somnifera improves semen quali-ty by regulating reproductive hormone levels and oxidative stress in seminal plasma of infertile males. *Fertil Steril.* 2010 Aug;94(3):989-96.

601   Bhattacharya SK, Muruganandam AV. Adaptogenic activity of Withania somnifera: an experimental study using a rat model of chronic stress. *Pharmacol Biochem Behav.* 2003 Jun;75(3):547-55.

602   Bhattacharya SK, Bhattacharya A, Sairam K, Ghosal S. Anxiolytic-antidepressant activity of Withania somnifera glycowithanolides: an experimental study. *Phytomedi-cine.* 2000 Dec;7(6):463-9.

603   Bone K. Clinical Applications of Ayurvedic and Chinese Herbs. Monographs for the Western Herbal Practitioner. Australia: Phytotherapy Press;1996:137-141.

604   Mayola E, Gallerne C, Esposti DD, et al. Withaferin A induces apoptosis in human melanoma cells through generation of reactive oxygen species and down-regulation of Bcl-2. *Apoptosis.* 2011 Oct;16(10):1014-27.

605   Sehgal N, Gupta A, Valli RK, et al. Withania somnifera reverses Alzheimer's disease pathology by enhancing low-density lipoprotein receptor-related protein in liver. *Proc Natl Acad Sci U S A.* 2012;109(9):3510-5.

606   Ahmad MK, Mahdi AA, Shukla KK, et al. Withania somnifera improves semen quali-ty by regulating reproductive hormone levels and oxidative stress in seminal plasma of infertile males. *Fertil Steril.* 2010 Aug;94(3):989-96.

607   Gupta GL, Rana AC. Protective effect of Withania somnifera dunal root extract against protracted social isolation induced behavior in rats. *Indian J Physiol Pharmacol.*

2007 Oct-Dec;51(4):345-53.

608   Bhattacharya SK, Bhattacharya A, Sairam K, Ghosal S. Anxiolytic-antidepressant activity of Withania somnifera glycowithanolides: an experimental study. *Phytomedicine*. 2000 Dec;7(6):463-9.

609   Kumar A, Kalonia H. Effect of Withania somnifera on Sleep-Wake Cycle in Sleep-Disturbed Rats: Possible GABAergic Mechanism. *Indian J Pharm Sci.* 2008 Nov;70(6):806-10.

610   Naidu PS, Singh A, Kulkarni SK. Effect of Withania somnifera root extract on reserpine-induced orofacial dyskinesia and cognitive dysfunction. *Phytother Res.* 2006 Feb;20(2):140-6.

611   Gupta GL, Rana AC. Effect of Withania somnifera Dunal in ethanol-induced anxiolysis and withdrawal anxiety in rats. *Indian J Exp Biol.* 2008 Jun;46(6):470-5.

612   Soman S, Korah PK, Jayanarayanan S, Mathew J, Paulose CS. Oxidative stress induced NMDA receptor alteration leads to spatial memory deficits in temporal lobe epilepsy: ameliorative effects of Withania somnifera and Withanolide A. *Neurochem Res.* 2012 Sep;37(9):1915-27. doi: 10.1007/s11064-012-0810-5.

613   Ilayperuma I, Ratnasooriya WD, Weerasooriya TR. Effect of Withania somnifera root extract on the sexual behaviour of male rats. *Asian J Androl.* 2002 Dec;4(4):295-8.

614   RajaSankar S, Manivasagam T, Sankar V, et al. Withania somnifera root extract improves catecholamines and physiological abnormalities seen in a Parkinson's disease model mouse. *J Ethnopharmacol.* 2009 Sep 25;125(3):369-73. doi: 10.1016/j.jep.2009.08.003.

615   Kulkarni SK, Akula KK, Dhir A. Effect of Withania somnifera Dunal root extract against pentylenetetrazol seizure threshold in mice: possible involvement of GABAergic system. *Indian J Exp Biol.* 2008 Jun;46(6):465-9.

616   Schliebs R, Liebmann A, Bhattacharya SK, Kumar A, Ghosal S, Bigl V. Systemic administration of defined extracts from Withania somnifera (Indian Ginseng) and Shilajit differentially affects cholinergic but not glutamatergic and GABAergic markers in rat brain. *Neurochem Int.* 1997 Feb;30(2):181-90.

617   Sehgal N, Gupta A, Valli RK, et al. Withania somnifera reverses Alzheimer's disease pathology by enhancing low-density lipoprotein receptor-related protein in liver. *Proc Natl Acad Sci U S A.* 2012; 109(9):3510-5.

618   Abdel-Magied EM, Abdel-Rahman HA, Harraz FM. The effect of aqueous extracts of Cynomorium coccineum and Withania somnifera on testicular development in immature Wistar rats. *J Ethnopharmacol.* 2001 Apr;75(1):1-4.

619   Abdel-Magied EM, Abdel-Rahman HA, Harraz FM. The effect of aqueous extracts of Cynomorium coccineum and Withania somnifera on testicular development in immature Wistar rats. *J Ethnopharmacol.* 2001 Apr;75(1):1-4.

620   Al-Qarawi AA, Abdel-Rahman HA, El-Badry AA, Harraz F, Razig NA, Abdel-Magied EM. The effect of extracts of Cynomorium coccineum and Withania somnifera on gonadotrophins and ovarian follicles of immature Wistar rats. *Phytother Res.* 2000 Jun;14(4):288-90.

621   Mahdi AA, Shukla KK, Ahmad MK, et al. Withania somnifera improves semen quality in stress-related male fertility. *Evid Based Complement Alternat Med.*

2011;2011:576962.

622   Sehgal N, Gupta A, Valli RK, et al. Withania somnifera reverses Alzheimer's disease pathology by enhancing low-density lipoprotein receptor-related protein in liver. *Proc Natl Acad Sci U S A.* 2012;109(9):3510-5.

623   Sehgal N, Gupta A, Valli RK, et al. Withania somnifera reverses Alzheimer's disease pathology by enhancing low-density lipoprotein receptor-related protein in liver. *Proc Natl Acad Sci U S A.* 2012;109(9):3510-5.

624   Ilayperuma I, Ratnasooriya WD, Weerasooriya TR. Effect of Withania somnifera root extract on the sexual behaviour of male rats. *Asian J Androl.* 2002 Dec;4(4):295-8.

625   Abdel-Magied EM, Abdel-Rahman HA, Harraz FM. The effect of aqueous extracts of Cynomorium coccineum and Withania somnifera on testicular development in immature Wistar rats. *J Ethnopharmacol.* 2001 Apr;75(1):1-4.

626   Andrade C, Aswath A, Chaturvedi SK, Srinivasa M, Raguram R. A double-blind, placebo-controlled evaluation of the anxiolytic efficacy of an ethanolic extract of withania somnifera. *Indian J Psychiatry.* 2000 Jul;42(3):295-301.

627   Sehgal N, Gupta A, Valli RK, et al. Withania somnifera reverses Alzheimer's disease pathology by enhancing low-density lipoprotein receptor-related protein in liver. *Proc Natl Acad Sci U S A.* 2012;109(9):3510-5.

628   Sehgal N, Gupta A, Valli RK, et al. Withania somnifera reverses Alzheimer's disease pathology by enhancing low-density lipoprotein receptor-related protein in liver. *Proc Natl Acad Sci U S A.* 2012;109(9):3510-5.

629   Sehgal N, Gupta A, Valli RK, et al. Withania somnifera reverses Alzheimer's disease pathology by enhancing low-density lipoprotein receptor-related protein in liver. *Proc Natl Acad Sci U S A.* 2012;109(9):3510-5.

630   Van der Hooft CS, Hoekstra A, Winter A, de Smet PA, Stricker BH. Thyrotoxicosis following the use of ashwagandha. *Ned Tijdschr Geneeskd.* 2005 Nov 19;149(47):2637-8.

631   Sehgal N, Gupta A, Valli RK, et al. Withania somnifera reverses Alzheimer's disease pathology by enhancing low-density lipoprotein receptor-related protein in liver. *Proc Natl Acad Sci U S A.* 2012;109(9):3510-5.

632   Gohil KJ, Patel JA, Gajjar AK. Pharmacological Review on Centella asiatica: A Potential Herbal Cure-all. *Indian J Pharm Sci.* 2010 Sep;72(5):546-56. doi: 10.4103/0250-474X.78519.

633   Orhan IE. Centella asiatica (L.) Urban: From Traditional Medicine to Modern Medicine with Neuroprotective Potential. *Evid Based Complement Alternat Med.* 2012;2012:946259. doi: 10.1155/2012/946259.

634   Pittella F, Dutra RC, Junior DD, Lopes MT, Barbosa NR. Antioxidant and cytotoxic activities of Centella asiatica (L) Urb. *Int J Mol Sci.* 2009 Aug 26;10(9):3713-21. doi: 10.3390/ijms10093713.

635   Pittella F, Dutra RC, Junior DD, Lopes MT, Barbosa NR. Antioxidant and cytotoxic activities of Centella asiatica (L) Urb. *Int J Mol Sci.* 2009 Aug 26;10(9):3713-21. doi: 10.3390/ijms10093713.

636   Pittella F, Dutra RC, Junior DD, Lopes MT, Barbosa NR. Antioxidant and cytotox-

ic activities of Centella asiatica (L) Urb. *Int J Mol Sci.* 2009 Aug 26;10(9):3713-21. doi: 10.3390/ijms10093713.

637   Pittella F, Dutra RC, Junior DD, Lopes MT, Barbosa NR. Antioxidant and cytotoxic activities of Centella asiatica (L) Urb. *Int J Mol Sci.* 2009 Aug 26;10(9):3713-21. doi: 10.3390/ijms10093713.

638   Di Paola R, Esposito E, Mazzon E, et al. 3,5-Dicaffeoyl-4-malonylquinic acid reduced oxidative stress and inflammation in a experimental model of inflammatory bowel disease. *Free Radic Res.* 2010 Jan;44(1):74-89. doi: 10.3109/10715760903300709.

639   Centella asiatica. *Altern Med Rev.* 2007 Mar;12(1):69-72.

640   Pittella F, Dutra RC, Junior DD, Lopes MT, Barbosa NR. Antioxidant and cytotoxic activities of Centella asiatica (L) Urb. *Int J Mol Sci.* 2009 Aug 26;10(9):3713-21. doi: 10.3390/ijms10093713.

641   Visweswari G, Prasad KS, Chetan PS, Lokanatha V, Rajendra W. Evaluation of the anticonvulsant effect of Centella asiatica (gotu kola) in pentylenetetrazol-induced seizures with respect to cholinergic neurotransmission. *Epilepsy Behav.* 2010 Mar;17(3):332-5. doi: 10.1016/j.yebeh.2010.01.002.

642   Kumar A, Dogra S, Prakash A. Neuroprotective effects of Centella asiatica against intracerebroventricular colchicine-induced cognitive impairment and oxidative stress. *Int J Alzheimers Dis.* 2009;2009:972178.

643   Centella asiatica. *Altern Med Rev.* 2007 Mar;12(1):69-72.

644   Awad R, Levac D, Cybulska P, Merali Z, Trudeau VL, Arnason JT. Effects of traditionally used anxiolytic botanicals on enzymes of the gamma-aminobutyric acid (GABA) system. *Can J Physiol Pharmacol.* 2007 Sep;85(9):933-42.

645   Centella asiatica. *Altern Med Rev.* 2007 Mar;12(1):69-72.

646   Centella asiatica. *Altern Med Rev.* 2007 Mar;12(1):69-72.

647   Prakash A, Kumar A. Mitoprotective effect of Centella asiatica against aluminum-induced neurotoxicity in rats: possible relevance to its anti-oxidant and anti-apoptosis mechanism. *Neurol Sci.* 2013;34(8):1403-9.

648   Centella asiatica. *Altern Med Rev.* 2007 Mar;12(1):69-72.

649   Centella asiatica. *Altern Med Rev.* 2007 Mar;12(1):69-72.

650   Centella asiatica. *Altern Med Rev.* 2007 Mar;12(1):69-72.

651   Dhanasekaran M, Holcomb LA, Hitt AR, et al. Centella asiatica extract selectively decreases amyloid beta levels in hippocampus of Alzheimer's disease animal model. *Phytother Res.* 2009 Jan;23(1):14-9. doi: 10.1002/ptr.2405.

652   Katz M, Levine AA, Kol-Degani H, Kav-Venaki L. A compound herbal preparation (CHP) in the treatment of children with ADHD: a randomized controlled trial. *J Atten Disord.* 2010 Nov;14(3):281-91. doi: 10.1177/1087054709356388.

653   Centella asiatica. *Altern Med Rev.* 2007 Mar;12(1):69-72.

654   Wattanathorn J, Mator L, Muchimapura S, et al. Positive modulation of cognition and mood in the healthy elderly volunteer following the administration of Centella asiatica. *J Ethnopharmacol.* 2008 Mar 5;116(2):325-32. doi: 10.1016/j.jep.2007.11.038.

655   Yunianto I, Das S, Mat Noor M. Antispermatogenic and antifertility effect of Pegaga

(Centella asiatica L) on the testis of male Sprague-Dawley rats. *Clin Ter.* 2010;161(3):235-9.

656   Centella asiatica. *Altern Med Rev.* 2007 Mar;12(1):69-72.

657   Pan Y, Abd-Rashid BA, Ismail Z, et al. In vitro modulatory effects on three major human cytochrome P450 enzymes by multiple active constituents and extracts of Centella asiatica. *J Ethnopharmacol.* 2010 Jul 20;130(2):275-83. doi: 10.1016/j. jep.2010.05.002.

658   Centella asiatica. *Altern Med Rev.* 2007 Mar;12(1):69-72.

659   Jorge OA, Jorge AD. Hepatotoxicity associated with the ingestion of Centella asiatica. *Rev Esp Enferm Dig.* 2005 Feb;97(2):115-24.

660   Centella asiatica. *Altern Med Rev.* 2007 Mar;12(1):69-72.

661   Centella asiatica. *Altern Med Rev.* 2007 Mar;12(1):69-72.

662   Centella asiatica. *Altern Med Rev.* 2007 Mar;12(1):69-72.

663   Centella asiatica. *Altern Med Rev.* 2007 Mar;12(1):69-72.

664   Kulshreshtha A, Zacharia AJ, Jarouliya U, Bhadauriya P, Prasad GB, Bisen PS. Spirulina in health care management. *Curr Pharm Biotechnol.* 2008 Oct;9(5):400-5.

665   Yang HN, Lee EH, Kim HM. Spirulina platensis inhibits anaphylactic reaction. *Life Sci.* 1997;61(13):1237-44.

666   Yang HN, Lee EH, Kim HM. Spirulina platensis inhibits anaphylactic reaction. *Life Sci.* 1997;61(13):1237-44.

667   Yang HN, Lee EH, Kim HM. Spirulina platensis inhibits anaphylactic reaction. *Life Sci.* 1997;61(13):1237-44.

668   Kim NH, Jeong HJ, Lee JY, et al. The effect of hydrolyzed Spirulina by malted barley on forced swimming test in ICR mice. *Int J Neurosci.* 2008 Nov;118(11):1523-33. doi: 10.1080/00207450802325603.

669   Thaakur SR, Jyothi B. Effect of spirulina maxima on the haloperidol induced tardive dyskinesia and oxidative stress in rats. *J Neural Transm.* 2007 Sep;114(9):1217-25.

670   Yang HN, Lee EH, Kim HM. Spirulina platensis inhibits anaphylactic reaction. *Life Sci.* 1997;61(13):1237-44.

671   Yang HN, Lee EH, Kim HM. Spirulina platensis inhibits anaphylactic reaction. *Life Sci.* 1997;61(13):1237-44.

672   Kim HM, Lee EH, Cho HH, Moon YH. Inhibitory effect of mast cell-mediated immediate-type allergic reactions in rats by spirulina. *Biochem Pharmacol.* 1998 Apr 1;55(7):1071-6.

673   Mao TK, Van de Water J, Gershwin ME. Effects of a Spirulina-based dietary supplement on cytokine production from allergic rhinitis patients. *J Med Food.* 2005 Spring;8(1):27-30.

674   Cingi C, Conk-Dalay M, Cakli H, Bal C. The effects of spirulina on allergic rhinitis. *Eur Arch Otorhinolaryngol.* 2008 Oct;265(10):1219-23. doi: 10.1007/s00405-008-0642-8.

675   Sharoba, Ashraf. Nutritional value of spirulina and its use in the preparation

of some complementary baby food formulas. Agroalimentary Processes and Technologies. 2014 20(4), 330-350.

676   U.S. Food and Drug Administration website. http://www.fda.gov/downloads/Food/IngredientsPackagingLabeling/GRAS/NoticeInventory/UCM265861#page=1&zoom=auto,-55,805

677   Bacopa monniera. Monograph. *Altern Med Rev.* 2004 Mar;9(1):79-85.

678   Bacopa monniera. Monograph. *Altern Med Rev.* 2004 Mar;9(1):79-85.

679   Rajan KE, Singh HK, Parkavi A, Charles PD. Attenuation of 1-(m-chloro-phenyl)-biguanide induced hippocampus-dependent memory impairment by a standardised extract of Bacopa monniera (BESEB CDRI-08). *Neurochem Res.* 2011 Nov;36(11):2136-44. doi: 10.1007/s11064-011-0538-7.

680   Tripathi S, Mahdi AA, Hasan M, Mitra K, Mahdi F. Protective potential of Bacopa monniera (Brahmi) extract on aluminum induced cerebellar toxicity and associated neuromuscular status in aged rats. *Cell Mol Biol (Noisy-le-grand).* 2011 Feb 12;57(1):3-15.

681   Charles PD, Ambigapathy G, Geraldine P, Akbarsha MA, Rajan KE. Bacopa monniera leaf extract up-regulates tryptophan hydroxylase (TPH2) and serotonin transporter (SERT) expression: implications in memory formation. *J Ethnopharmacol.* 2011 Mar 8;134(1):55-61. doi: 10.1016/j.jep.2010.11.045.

682   Sheikh N, Ahmad A, Siripurapu KB, Kuchibhotla VK, Singh S, Palit G. Effect of Bacopa monniera on stress induced changes in plasma corticosterone and brain mono-amines in rats. *J Ethnopharmacol.* 2007 May 22;111(3):671-6.

683   Lohidasan S, Paradkar AR, Mahadik KR. Nootropic activity of lipid-based extract of Bacopa monniera Linn. compared with traditional preparation and extracts. *J Pharm Pharmacol.* 2009 Nov;61(11):1537-44. doi: 10.1211/jpp.61.11.0014.

684   Mathew J, Balakrishnan S, Antony S, Abraham PM, Paulose CS. Decreased GABA receptor in the cerebral cortex of epileptic rats: effect of Bacopa monnieri and Baco-side-A. *J Biomed Sci.* 2012 Feb 24;19:25. doi: 10.1186/1423-0127-19-25.

685   Mathew J, Balakrishnan S, Antony S, Abraham PM, Paulose CS. Decreased GABA receptor in the cerebral cortex of epileptic rats: effect of Bacopa monnieri and Baco-side-A. *J Biomed Sci.* 2012 Feb 24;19:25. doi: 10.1186/1423-0127-19-25.

686   Lohidasan S, Paradkar AR, Mahadik KR. Nootropic activity of lipid-based extract of Bacopa monniera Linn. compared with traditional preparation and extracts. *J Pharm Pharmacol.* 2009 Nov;61(11):1537-44. doi: 10.1211/jpp.61.11.0014.

687   Khan R, Krishnakumar A, Paulose CS. Decreased glutamate receptor binding and NMDA R1 gene expression in hippocampus of pilocarpine-induced epileptic rats: neuro-protective role of Bacopa monnieri extract. *Epilepsy Behav.* 2008 Jan;12(1):54-60.

688   Mathew J, Balakrishnan S, Antony S, Abraham PM, Paulose CS. Decreased GABA receptor in the cerebral cortex of epileptic rats: effect of Bacopa monnieri and Baco-side-A. *J Biomed Sci.* 2012 Feb 24;19:25. doi: 10.1186/1423-0127-19-25.

689   Prabhakar S, Saraf MK, Pandhi P, Anand A. Bacopa monniera exerts antiamnesic effect on diazepam-induced anterograde amnesia in mice. *Psychopharmacology (Berl).* 2008 Sep;200(1):27-37. doi: 10.1007/s00213-007-1049-8.

690   Negi KS, Singh YD, Kushwaha KP, et al. Clinical evaluation of memory enhancing properties of memory plus in children with attention deficit hyperactivity disorder. *Indian J Psychiatry.* 2000; 42(2) Supplement.

691   Mathew J, Balakrishnan S, Antony S, Abraham PM, Paulose CS. Decreased GABA receptor in the cerebral cortex of epileptic rats: effect of Bacopa monnieri and Baco-side-A. *J Biomed Sci.* 2012 Feb 24;19:25. doi: 10.1186/1423-0127-19-25.

692   Chatterjee M, Verma P, Palit G. Comparative evaluation of Bacopa monniera and Panax quniquefolium in experimental anxiety and depressive models in mice. *Indian J Exp Biol.* 2010 Mar;48(3):306-13.

693   Bhattacharya SK, Ghosal S. Anxiolytic activity of a standardized extract of Bacopa monniera: an experimental study. *Phytomedicine.* 1998 Apr;5(2):77-82. doi: 10.1016/S0944-7113(98)80001-9.

694   Pase MP, Kean J, Sarris J, Neale C, Scholey AB, Stough C. The cognitive-enhancing effects of Bacopa monnieri: a systematic review of randomized, controlled human clinical trials. *J Altern Complement Med.* 2012 Jul;18(7):647-52. doi: 10.1089/acm.2011.0367.

695   Sairam K, Dorababu M, Goel RK, Bhattacharya SK. Antidepressant activity of standardized extract of Bacopa monniera in experimental models of depression in rats. *Phytomedicine.* 2002 Apr;9(3):207-11.

696   Mathew J, Balakrishnan S, Antony S, Abraham PM, Paulose CS. Decreased GABA receptor in the cerebral cortex of epileptic rats: effect of Bacopa monnieri and Baco-side-A. *J Biomed Sci.* 2012 Feb 24;19:25. doi: 10.1186/1423-0127-19-25.

697   Negi KS, Singh YD, Kushwaha KP, et al. Clinical evaluation of memory enhancing properties of memory plus in children with attention deficit hyperactivity disorder. *Indian J Psychiatry.* 2000;42(2)suppl.

698   Usha PD, Wasim P, Joshua JA, et al. BacoMind®: A Cognitive Enhancer in Children Requiring Individual Education Programme. *J Pharm Tox.* 2008;3:302-310.

699   Pase MP, Kean J, Sarris J, Neale C, Scholey AB, Stough C. The cognitive-en-hancing effects of Bacopa monnieri: a systematic review of randomized, controlled human clinical trials. *J Altern Complement Med.* 2012 Jul;18(7):647-52. doi: 10.1089/acm.2011.0367.

700   Sathyanarayanan V, Thomas T, Einöther SJ, Dobriyal R, Joshi MK, Krishnam-achari S. Brahmi for the better? New findings challenging cognition and anti-anxiety effects of Brahmi (Bacopa monniera) in healthy adults. *Psychopharmacology (Berl).* 2013;227(2):299-306.

701   Singh A, Singh SK. Evaluation of antifertility potential of Brahmi in male mouse. *Contraception.* 2009 Jan;79(1):71-9. doi: 10.1016/j.contraception.2008.07.023.

702   Mathew J, Balakrishnan S, Antony S, Abraham PM, Paulose CS. Decreased GABA receptor in the cerebral cortex of epileptic rats: effect of Bacopa monnieri and Baco-side-A. *J Biomed Sci.* 2012 Feb 24;19:25. doi: 10.1186/1423-0127-19-25.

703   Mathew J, Balakrishnan S, Antony S, Abraham PM, Paulose CS. Decreased GABA receptor in the cerebral cortex of epileptic rats: effect of Bacopa monnieri and Baco-side-A. *J Biomed Sci.* 2012 Feb 24;19:25. doi: 10.1186/1423-0127-19-25.

Notes

704   Pravina K, Ravindra KR, Goudar KS, et al. Safety evaluation of BacoMind in healthy volunteers: a phase I study. *Phytomedicine.* 2007 May;14(5):301-8.

705   Joshua Allan J, Damodaran A, Deshmukh NS, Goudar KS, Amit A. Safety evaluation of a standardized phytochemical composition extracted from Bacopa monnieri in Sprague--Dawley rats. *Food Chem Toxicol.* 2007 Oct;45(10):1928-37.

706   Pravina K, Ravindra KR, Goudar KS, et al. Safety evaluation of BacoMind in healthy volunteers: a phase I study. *Phytomedicine.* 2007 May;14(5):301-8.

707   Mathew J, Balakrishnan S, Antony S, Abraham PM, Paulose CS. Decreased GABA receptor in the cerebral cortex of epileptic rats: effect of Bacopa monnieri and Bacoside-A. *J Biomed Sci.* 2012 Feb 24;19:25. doi: 10.1186/1423-0127-19-25.

708   Lemon balm. University of Maryland Medical Center website. http://umm.edu/health/medical/altmed/herb/lemon-balm.

709   De Carvalho NC, Corrêa-Angeloni MJ, Leffa DD, et al. Evaluation of the genotoxic and antigenotoxic potential of Melissa officinalis in mice. *Genet Mol Biol.* 2011 Apr;34(2):290-7.

710   Chung MJ, Cho SY, Bhuiyan MJ, Kim KH, Lee SJ. Anti-diabetic effects of lemon balm (Melissa officinalis) essential oil on glucose- and lipid-regulating enzymes in type 2 diabetic mice. *Br J Nutr.* 2010 Jul;104(2):180-8. doi: 10.1017/S0007114510001765.

711   Guginski G, Luiz AP, Silva MD, et al. Mechanisms involved in the antinociception caused by ethanolic extract obtained from the leaves of Melissa officinalis (lemon balm) in mice. *Pharmacol Biochem Behav.* 2009 Jul;93(1):10-6. doi: 10.1016/j.pbb.2009.03.014.

712   De Sousa AC, Alviano DS, Blank AF, Alves PB, Alviano CS, Gattass CR. Melissa officinalis L. essential oil: antitumoral and antioxidant activities. *J Pharm Pharmacol.* 2004 May;56(5):677-81.

713   Mazzanti G, Battinelli L, Pompeo C, et al. Inhibitory activity of Melissa officinalis L. extract on Herpes simplex virus type 2 replication. *Nat Prod Res.* 2008;22(16):1433-40. doi: 10.1080/14786410802075939.

714   Hăncianu M, Aprotosoaie AC, Gille E, et al. Chemical composition and in vitro antimicrobial activity of essential oil of Melissa officinalis L. from Romania. *Rev Med Chir Soc Med Nat Iasi.* 2008 Jul-Sep;112(3):843-7.

715   Yoo DY, Choi JH, Kim W, et al. Effects of Melissa officinalis L. (lemon balm) extract on neurogenesis associated with serum corticosterone and GABA in the mouse dentate gyrus. *Neurochem Res.* 2011 Feb;36(2):250-7. doi: 10.1007/s11064-010-0312-2.

716   De Carvalho NC, Corrêa-Angeloni MJ, Leffa DD, et al. Evaluation of the genotoxic and antigenotoxic potential of Melissa officinalis in mice. *Genet Mol Biol.* 2011 Apr;34(2):290-7.

717   Mimica-Dukic N, Bozin B, Sokovic M, Simin N. Antimicrobial and antioxidant activities of Melissa officinalis L. (Lamiaceae) essential oil. *J Agric Food Chem.* 2004 May 5;52(9):2485-9.

718   Zeraatpishe A, Oryan S, Bagheri MH, et al. Effects of Melissa officinalis L. on oxidative status and DNA damage in subjects exposed to long-term low-dose ionizing radiation. *Toxicol Ind Health.* 2011 Apr;27(3):205-12. doi: 10.1177/0748233710383889.

719   Awad R, Muhammad A, Durst T, Trudeau VL, Arnason JT. Bioassay-guided fractionation of lemon balm (Melissa officinalis L.) using an in vitro measure of GABA transaminase activity. *Phytother Res.* 2009 Aug;23(8):1075-81. doi: 10.1002/ptr.2712.

720   Cases J, Ibarra A, Feuillère N, Roller M, Sukkar SG. Pilot trial of Melissa officinalis L. leaf extract in the treatment of volunteers suffering from mild-to-moderate anxiety disorders and sleep disturbances. *Med J Nutrition Metab.* 2011 Dec;4(3):211-218.

721   Kennedy DO, Little W, Scholey AB. Attenuation of laboratory-induced stress in humans after acute administration of Melissa officinalis (Lemon Balm). *Psychosom Med.* 2004 Jul-Aug;66(4):607-13.

722   Yoo DY, Choi JH, Kim W, et al. Effects of Melissa officinalis L. (lemon balm) extract on neurogenesis associated with serum corticosterone and GABA in the mouse dentate gyrus. *Neurochem Res.* 2011 Feb;36(2):250-7. doi: 10.1007/s11064-010-0312-2.

723   Kennedy DO, Wake G, Savelev S, et al. Modulation of mood and cognitive performance following acute administration of single doses of Melissa officinalis (Lemon balm) with human CNS nicotinic and muscarinic receptor-binding properties. *Neuropsychopharmacology.* 2003 Oct;28(10):1871-81.

724   Müller SF, Klement S. A combination of valerian and lemon balm is effective in the treatment of restlessness and dyssomnia in children. *Phytomedicine.* 2006 Jun;13(6):383-7.

725   US Food and Drug Administration Website. https://www.accessdata.fda.gov/scripts/cdrh/cfdocs/cfcfr/cfrsearch.cfm?cfrpart=182&showfr=1. August 21, 2015.

726   Yoo DY, Choi JH, Kim W, et al. Effects of Melissa officinalis L. (lemon balm) extract on neurogenesis associated with serum corticosterone and GABA in the mouse dentate gyrus. *Neurochem Res.* 2011 Feb;36(2):250-7. doi: 10.1007/s11064-010-0312-2.

727   Yoo DY, Choi JH, Kim W, et al. Effects of Melissa officinalis L. (lemon balm) extract on neurogenesis associated with serum corticosterone and GABA in the mouse dentate gyrus. *Neurochem Res.* 2011 Feb;36(2):250-7. doi: 10.1007/s11064-010-0312-2.

728   De Carvalho NC, Corrêa-Angeloni MJ, Leffa DD, et al. Evaluation of the genotoxic and antigenotoxic potential of Melissa officinalis in mice. *Genet Mol Biol.* 2011 Apr;34(2):290-7.

729   Srivastava JK, Shankar E, Gupta S. Chamomile: An Herbal Medicine of the Past with a Bright Future. Mol Med Rep. 2010 Nov 1;3(6):895-901.

730   Matricaria chamomilla (German chamomile). Monograph. *Altern Med Rev.* 2008 Mar;13(1):58-62.

731   Zanoli P, Avallone R, Baraldi M. Behavioral characterisation of the flavonoids apigenin and chrysin. *Fitoterapia.* 2000 Aug;71 Suppl 1:S117-23.

732   Zanoli P, Avallone R, Baraldi M. Behavioral characterisation of the flavonoids apigenin and chrysin. *Fitoterapia.* 2000 Aug;71 Suppl 1:S117-23.

733   Chandrashekhar VM, Halagali KS, Nidavani RB, et al. Anti-allergic activity of German chamomile (Matricaria recutita L.) in mast cell mediated allergy model. *J Ethnopharmacol.* 2011 Sep 1;137(1):336-40. doi: 10.1016/j.jep.2011.05.029.

734   Guimarães R, Barros L, Dueñas M, et al. Infusion and decoction of wild German chamomile: bioactivity and characterization of organic acids and phenolic compounds. *Food Chem.* 2013 Jan 15;136(2):947-54. doi: 10.1016/j.foodchem.2012.09.007.

Notes

735   Awad R, Levac D, Cybulska P, Merali Z, Trudeau VL, Arnason JT. Effects of traditionally used anxiolytic botanicals on enzymes of the gamma-aminobutyric acid (GABA) system. *Can J Physiol Pharmacol.* 2007 Sep;85(9):933-42.

736   Kim JW, Kim CS, Hu Z, et al. Enhancement of pentobarbital-induced sleep by apigenin through chloride ion channel activation. *Arch Pharm Res.* 2012 Feb;35(2):367-73. doi: 10.1007/s12272-012-0218-4.

737   Zanoli P, Avallone R, Baraldi M. Behavioral characterisation of the flavonoids apigenin and chrysin. *Fitoterapia.* 2000 Aug;71 Suppl 1:S117-23.

738   Viola H, Wasowski C, Levi de Stein M, et al. Apigenin, a component of Matricaria recutita flowers, is a central benzodiazepine receptors-ligand with anxiolytic effects. *Planta Med.* 1995 Jun;61(3):213-6.

739   Nakazawa T, Yasuda T, Ueda J, Ohsawa K. Antidepressant-like effects of apigenin and 2,4,5-trimethoxycinnamic acid from Perilla frutescens in the forced swimming test. *Biol Pharm Bull.* 2003 Apr;26(4):474-80.

740   Nakazawa T, Yasuda T, Ueda J, Ohsawa K. Antidepressant-like effects of apigenin and 2,4,5-trimethoxycinnamic acid from Perilla frutescens in the forced swimming test. *Biol Pharm Bull.* 2003 Apr;26(4):474-80.

741   Campbell EL, Chebib M, Johnston GA. The dietary flavonoids apigenin and (-)-epigallocatechin gallate enhance the positive modulation by diazepam of the activation by GABA of recombinant GABA(A) receptors. *Biochem Pharmacol.* 2004 Oct 15;68(8):1631-8.

742   Yi LT, Li JM, Li YC, Pan Y, Xu Q, Kong LD. Antidepressant-like behavioral and neurochemical effects of the citrus-associated chemical apigenin. *Life Sci.* 2008 Mar 26;82(13-14):741-51. doi: 10.1016/j.lfs.2008.01.007.

743   Zhao G, Qin GW, Wang J, Chu WJ, Guo LH. Functional activation of monoamine transporters by luteolin and apigenin isolated from the fruit of Perilla frutescens (L.) *Britt Neurochem Int.* 2010 Jan;56(1):168-76. doi: 10.1016/j.neuint.2009.09.015.

744   Nakazawa T, Yasuda T, Ueda J, Ohsawa K. Antidepressant-like effects of apigenin and 2,4,5-trimethoxycinnamic acid from Perilla frutescens in the forced swimming test. *Biol Pharm Bull.* 2003 Apr;26(4):474-80.

745   Han XH, Hong SS, Hwang JS, Lee MK, Hwang BY, Ro JS. Monoamine oxidase inhibitory components from Cayratia japonica. *Arch Pharm Res.* 2007 Jan;30(1):13-7.

746   Han JH, Kim KJ, Jang HJ, et al. Effects of Apigenin on Glutamate-induced [Ca] (i) Increases in Cultured Rat Hippocampal Neurons. *Korean J Physiol Pharmacol.* 2008 Apr;12(2):43-9. doi: 10.4196/kjpp.2008.12.2.43.

747   Shinomiya K, Inoue T, Utsu Y, et al. Hypnotic activities of chamomile and passiflora extracts in sleep-disturbed rats. *Biol Pharm Bull.* 2005 May;28(5):808-10.

748   Shinomiya K, Inoue T, Utsu Y, et al. Hypnotic activities of chamomile and passiflora extracts in sleep-disturbed rats. *Biol Pharm Bull.* 2005 May;28(5):808-10.

749   Shinomiya K, Inoue T, Utsu Y, et al. Hypnotic activities of chamomile and passiflora extracts in sleep-disturbed rats. *Biol Pharm Bull.* 2005 May;28(5):808-10.

750   Losi G, Puia G, Garzon G, de Vuono MC, Baraldi M. Apigenin modulates GABAergic and glutamatergic transmission in cultured cortical neurons. *Eur J Pharmacol.* 2004 Oct 11;502(1-2):41-6.

751   Can OD, Demir Özkay U, Kıyan HT, Demirci B. Psychopharmacological profile of Chamomile (Matricaria recutita L.) essential oil in mice. *Phytomedicine*. 2012 Feb 15;19(3-4):306-10. doi: 10.1016/j.phymed.2011.10.001.

752   Zick SM, Wright BD, Sen A, Arnedt JT. Preliminary examination of the efficacy and safety of a standardized chamomile extract for chronic primary insomnia: a randomized placebo-controlled pilot study. *BMC Complement Altern Med*. 2011 Sep 22;11:78. doi: 10.1186/1472-6882-11-78.

753   Shinomiya K, Inoue T, Utsu Y, et al. Hypnotic activities of chamomile and passiflora extracts in sleep-disturbed rats. *Biol Pharm Bull*. 2005 May;28(5):808-10.

754   Amsterdam JD, Li Y, Soeller I, Rockwell K, Mao JJ, Shults J. A randomized, double-blind, placebo-controlled trial of oral Matricaria recutita (chamomile) extract therapy for generalized anxiety disorder. *J Clin Psychopharmacol*. 2009 Aug;29(4):378-82. doi: 10.1097/JCP.0b013e3181ac935c.

755   Amsterdam JD, Shults J, Soeller I, Mao JJ, Rockwell K, Newberg AB. Chamomile (Matricaria recutita) may provide antidepressant activity in anxious, depressed humans: an exploratory study. *Altern Ther Health Med*. 2012 Sep-Oct;18(5):44-9.

756   Niederhofer H. Observational study: Matricaria chamomilla may improve some symptoms of attention-deficit hyperactivity disorder. *Phytomedicine*. 2009 Apr;16(4):284-6. doi: 10.1016/j.phymed.2008.10.006.

757   Kim JW, Kim CS, Hu Z, et al. Enhancement of pentobarbital-induced sleep by apigenin through chloride ion channel activation. *Arch Pharm Res*. 2012 Feb;35(2):367-73. doi: 10.1007/s12272-012-0218-4.

758   Ogata I, Kawanai T, Hashimoto E, Nishimura Y, Oyama Y, Seo H. Bisabololoxide A, one of the main constituents in German chamomile extract, induces apoptosis in rat thymocytes. *Arch Toxicol*. 2010 Jan;84(1):45-52. doi: 10.1007/s00204-009-0472-5.

759   Ogata-Ikeda I, Seo H, Kawanai T, Hashimoto E, Oyama Y. Cytotoxic action of bisabololoxide A of German chamomile on human leukemia K562 cells in combination with 5-fluorouracil. *Phytomedicine*. 2011 Mar 15;18(5):362-5. doi: 10.1016/j.phymed.2010.08.007.

760   Kim JW, Kim CS, Hu Z, et al. Enhancement of pentobarbital-induced sleep by apigenin through chloride ion channel activation. *Arch Pharm Res*. 2012 Feb;35(2):367-73. doi: 10.1007/s12272-012-0218-4.

761   Appel K, Rose T, Fiebich B, Kammler T, Hoffmann C, Weiss G. Modulation of the γ-aminobutyric acid (GABA) system by Passiflora incarnata L. *Phytother Res*. 2011 Jun;25(6):838-43. doi: 10.1002/ptr.3352.

762   NYU Longane Medical Center website. Miroddi M, Calapai G, Navarra M, Minciullo PL, Gangemi S. Passiflora incarnata L.: ethnopharmacology, clinical application, safety and evaluation of clinical trials. *J Ethnopharmacol*. 2013 Dec 12;150(3):791-804. doi: 10.1016/j.jep.2013.09.047. Epub 2013 Oct 17.

763   Ulbricht C, Basch E, Boon H, et al. An evidence-based systematic review of passion flower (Passiflora incarnata L.) by the Natural Standard Research Collaboration. *J Diet Suppl*. 2008;5(3):310-40. doi: 10.1080/19390210802414360.

764   Breivogel C, Jamerson B. Passion flower extract antagonizes the expression of nicotine locomotor sensitization in rats. *Pharm Biol*. 2012 Oct;50(10):1310-6. doi: 10.3109/13880209.2012.674535.

Notes

765 CFR - Code of Federal Regulations Title 21. U.S. Food and Drug Administration website. https://www.accessdata.fda.gov/scripts/cdrh/cfdocs/cfcfr/CFRSearch. cfm?fr=172.510. Updated April 1, 2013.

766 Masteikova R, Bernatoniene J, Bernatoniene R, Velziene S. Antiradical activities of the extract of Passiflora incarnata. *Acta Pol Pharm.* 2008 Sep-Oct;65(5):577-83.

767 Gupta RK, Kumar D, Chaudhary AK, Maithani M, Singh R. Antidiabetic activity of Passiflora incarnata Linn. in streptozotocin-induced diabetes in mice. *J Ethnopharmacol.* 2012 Feb 15;139(3):801-6. doi: 10.1016/j.jep.2011.12.021.

768 Dhawan K, Kumar S, Sharma A. Antiasthmatic activity of the methanol extract of leaves of Passiflora incarnata. *Phytother Res.* 2003 Aug;17(7):821-2.

769 Breivogel C, Jamerson B. Passion flower extract antagonizes the expression of nicotine locomotor sensitization in rats. *Pharm Biol.* 2012 Oct;50(10):1310-6. doi: 10.3109/13880209.2012.674535.

770 Dhawan K, Sharma A. Antitussive activity of the methanol extract of Passiflora incarnata leaves. *Fitoterapia.* 2002 Aug;73(5):397-9.

771 Dhawan K, Kumar S, Sharma A. Antiasthmatic activity of the methanol extract of leaves of Passiflora incarnata. *Phytother Res.* 2003 Aug;17(7):821-2.

772 Dhawan K, Kumar S, Sharma A. Antiasthmatic activity of the methanol extract of leaves of Passiflora incarnata. *Phytother Res.* 2003 Aug;17(7):821-2.

773 Nassiri-Asl M, Zamansoltani F, Shariati-Rad S. Possible role of GABAA-benzodiazepine receptor in anticonvulsant effects of Pasipay in rats. *Zhong Xi Yi Jie He Xue Bao.* 2008 Nov;6(11):1170-3. doi: 10.3736/jcim20091112.

774 Nassiri-Asl M, Shariati-Rad S, Zamansoltani F. Anticonvulsant effects of aerial parts of Passiflora incarnata extract in mice: involvement of benzodiazepine and opioid receptors. *BMC Complement Altern Med.* 2007 Aug 8;7:26.

775 Grundmann O, Wähling C, Staiger C, Butterweck V. Anxiolytic effects of a passion flower (Passiflora incarnata L.) extract in the elevated plus maze in mice. *Pharmazie.* 2009 Jan;64(1):63-4.

776 Nassiri-Asl M, Zamansoltani F, Shariati-Rad S. Possible role of GABAA-benzodiazepine receptor in anticonvulsant effects of Pasipay in rats. *Zhong Xi Yi Jie He Xue Bao.* 2008 Nov;6(11):1170-3. doi: 10.3736/jcim20091112.

777 Nassiri-Asl M, Zamansoltani F, Shariati-Rad S. Possible role of GABAA-benzodiazepine receptor in anticonvulsant effects of Pasipay in rats. *Zhong Xi Yi Jie He Xue Bao.* 2008 Nov;6(11):1170-3. doi: 10.3736/jcim20091112.

778 Elsas SM, Rossi DJ, Raber J, et al. Passiflora incarnata L. (Passionflower) extracts elicit GABA currents in hippocampal neurons in vitro, and show anxiogenic and anticonvulsant effects in vivo, varying with extraction method. *Phytomedicine.* 2010 Oct;17(12):940-9. doi: 10.1016/j.phymed.2010.03.002.

779 Akhondzadeh S, Naghavi HR, Vazirian M, Shayeganpour A, Rashidi H, Khani M. Passionflower in the treatment of generalized anxiety: a pilot double-blind randomized controlled trial with oxazepam. *J Clin Pharm Ther.* 2001 Oct;26(5):363-7.

780 Dhawan K, Kumar S, Sharma A. Aphrodisiac activity of methanol extract of leaves of Passiflora incarnata Linn in mice. *Phytother Res.* 2003 Apr;17(4):401-3.

781   Aslanargun P, Cuvas O, Dikmen B, Aslan E, Yuksel MU. Passiflora incarnata Linneaus as an anxiolytic before spinal anesthesia. *J Anesth.* 2012 Feb;26(1):39-44. doi: 10.1007/s00540-011-1265-6.

782   Akhondzadeh S, Naghavi HR, Vazirian M, Shayeganpour A, Rashidi H, Khani M. Passionflower in the treatment of generalized anxiety: a pilot double-blind randomized controlled trial with oxazepam. *J Clin Pharm Ther.* 2001 Oct;26(5):363-7.

783   Ngan A, Conduit R. A double-blind, placebo-controlled investigation of the effects of Passiflora incarnata (passionflower) herbal tea on subjective sleep quality. *Phytother Res.* 2011 Aug;25(8):1153-9. doi: 10.1002/ptr.3400.

784   Akhondzadeh S, Kashani L, Mobaseri M, Hosseini SH, Nikzad S, Khani M. Passionflower in the treatment of opiates withdrawal: a double-blind randomized controlled trial. *J Clin Pharm Ther.* 2001 Oct;26(5):369-73.

785   Li HB, Ying XX, Lu J. The mechanism of vitexin-4''-O-glucoside protecting ECV-304 cells against tertbutyl hydroperoxide induced injury. *Nat Prod Res.* 2010 Nov;24(18):1695-703. doi: 10.1080/14786410902853847.

786   Dong L, Fan Y, Shao X, Chen Z. Vitexin protects against myocardial ischemia/ reperfusion injury in Langendorff-perfused rat hearts by attenuating inflammatory response and apoptosis. *Food Chem Toxicol.* 2011 Dec;49(12):3211-6. doi: 10.1016/j. fct.2011.09.040.

787   Yang SH, Liao PH, Pan YF, Chen SL, Chou SS, Chou MY. The novel p53-dependent metastatic and apoptotic pathway induced by vitexin in human oral cancer OC2 cells. *Phytother Res.* 2013;27(8):1154-61.

788   Dong LY, Chen ZW, Guo Y, Cheng XP, Shao X. Mechanisms of vitexin preconditioning effects on cultured neonatal rat cardiomyocytes with anoxia and reoxygenation. *Am J Chin Med.* 2008;36(2):385-97.

789   Demir Özkay U, Can OD. Anti-nociceptive effect of vitexin mediated by the opioid system in mice. *Pharmacol Biochem Behav.* 2013 Apr 30;109C:23-30. doi: 10.1016/j. pbb.2013.04.014.

790   Abbasi E, Nassiri-Asl M, Shafeei M, Sheikhi M. Neuroprotective effects of vitexin, a flavonoid, on pentylenetetrazole-induced seizure in rats. *Chem Biol Drug Des.* 2012 Aug;80(2):274-8. doi: 10.1111/j.1747-0285.2012.01400.x.

791   Can ÖD, Demir Özkay Ü, Üçel Uİ. Anti-depressant-like effect of vitexin in BALB/c mice and evidence for the involvement of monoaminergic mechanisms. *Eur J Pharmacol.* 2013 Jan 15;699(1-3):250-7. doi: 10.1016/j.ejphar.2012.10.017.

792   Abbasi E, Nassiri-Asl M, Sheikhi M, Shafiee M. Effects of vitexin on scopolamine-induced memory impairment in rats. *Chin J Physiol.* 2013;56(3):184-9.

793   Gaitan E, Cooksey RC, Legan J, Lindsay RH. Antithyroid effects in vivo and in vitro of vitexin: a C-glucosylflavone in millet. *J Clin Endocrinol Metab.* 1995 Apr;80(4):1144-7.

794   Gaitan E. Goitrogens in food and water. *Annu Rev Nutr.* 1990;10:21-39.

795   Wohlmuth H, Penman KG, Pearson T, Lehmann RP. Pharmacognosy and chemotypes of passionflower (Passiflora incarnata L.). *Biol Pharm Bull.* 2010;33(6):1015-8.

796   Lin CM, Huang ST, Liang YC, et al. Isovitexin suppresses lipopolysaccharide-mediated inducible nitric oxide synthase through inhibition of NF-kappa B in mouse macrophages. *Planta Med.* 2005 Aug;71(8):748-53.

Notes

797   Tse SY, Mak IT, Dickens BF. Antioxidative properties of harmane and beta-carboline alkaloids. *Biochem Pharmacol.* 1991 Jul 15;42(3):459-64.

798   Choo CY, Sulong NY, Man F, Wong TW. Vitexin and isovitexin from the Leaves of Ficus deltoidea with in-vivo α-glucosidase inhibition. *J Ethnopharmacol.* 2012 Aug 1;142(3):776-81. doi: 10.1016/j.jep.2012.05.062.

799   Zhai K, Hu L, Chen J, Fu CY, Chen Q. Chrysin induces hyperalgesia via the GABAA receptor in mice. *Planta Med.* 2008 Aug;74(10):1229-34. doi: 10.1055/s-2008-1081288.

800   Rashid S, Ali N, Nafees S, et al. Alleviation of doxorubicin-induced nephrotoxicity and hepatotoxicity by chrysin in Wistar rats. *Toxicol Mech Methods.* 2013;23(5):337-45.

801   Beaumont DM, Mark TM Jr, Hills R, Dixon P, Veit B, Garrett N. The effects of chrysin, a Passiflora incarnata extract, on natural killer cell activity in male Sprague-Dawley rats undergoing abdominal surgery. *AANA J.* 2008 Apr;76(2):113-7.

802   Medina JH, Paladini AC, Wolfman C, et al. Chrysin (5,7-di-OH-flavone), a naturally-occurring ligand for benzodiazepine receptors, with anticonvulsant properties. *Biochem Pharmacol.* 1990 Nov 15;40(10):2227-31.

803   Tse SY, Mak IT, Dickens BF. Antioxidative properties of harmane and beta-carboline alkaloids. *Biochem Pharmacol.* 1991 Jul 15;42(3):459-64.

804   Khan MS, Devaraj H, Devaraj N. Chrysin abrogates early hepatocarcinogenesis and induces apoptosis in N-nitrosodiethylamine-induced preneoplastic nodules in rats. *Toxicol Appl Pharmacol.* 2011 Feb 15;251(1):85-94. doi: 10.1016/j.taap.2010.12.004.

805   Zhai K, Hu L, Chen J, Fu CY, Chen Q. Chrysin induces hyperalgesia via the GABAA receptor in mice. *Planta Med.* 2008 Aug;74(10):1229-34. doi: 10.1055/s-2008-1081288.

806   Wolfman C, Viola H, Paladini A, Dajas F, Medina JH. Possible anxiolytic effects of chrysin, a central benzodiazepine receptor ligand isolated from Passiflora coerulea. *Pharmacol Biochem Behav.* 1994 Jan;47(1):1-4.

807   Tse SY, Mak IT, Dickens BF. Antioxidative properties of harmane and beta-carboline alkaloids. *Biochem Pharmacol.* 1991 Jul 15;42(3):459-64.

808   Brown E, Hurd NS, McCall S, Ceremuga TE. Evaluation of the anxiolytic effects of chrysin, a Passiflora incarnata extract, in the laboratory rat. *AANA J.* 2007 Oct;75(5):333-7.

809   Ergene E, Schoener EP. Effects of harmane (1-methyl-beta-carboline) on neurons in the nucleus accumbens of the rat. *Pharmacol Biochem Behav.* 1993 Apr;44(4):951-7.

810   Tsuji PA, Walle T. Cytotoxic effects of the dietary flavones chrysin and apigenin in a normal trout liver cell line. *Chem Biol Interact.* 2008 Jan 10;171(1):37-44.

811   Ta N, Walle T. Aromatase inhibition by bioavailable methylated flavones. *J Steroid Biochem Mol Biol.* 2007 Oct;107(1-2):127-9.

812   Tse SY, Mak IT, Dickens BF. Antioxidative properties of harmane and beta-carboline alkaloids. *Biochem Pharmacol.* 1991 Jul 15;42(3):459-64.

813   Ergene E, Schoener EP. Effects of harmane (1-methyl-beta-carboline) on neurons in the nucleus accumbens of the rat. *Pharmacol Biochem Behav.* 1993 Apr;44(4):951-7.

814   Louis ED, Benito-León J, Moreno-García S, et al. Blood harmane (1-methyl-9H-pyrido[3,4-b]indole) concentration in essential tremor cases in Spain. *Neurotoxicology.* 2013 Jan;34:264-8. doi: 10.1016/j.neuro.2012.09.004.

815   Abramets II, Komissarov IV. Ion-dependency of the GABA-potentiating effects of benzodiazepine tranquilizers and harmane. *Biull Eksp Biol Med.* 1984 Jun;97(6):679-81.

816   Singh B, Singh D, Goel RK. Dual protective effect of Passiflora incarnata in epilepsy and associated post-ictal depression. *J Ethnopharmacol.* 2012 Jan 6;139(1):273-9. doi: 10.1016/j.jep.2011.11.011.

817   Aricioglu F, Altunbas H. Harmane induces anxiolysis and antidepressant-like effects in rats. *Ann N Y Acad Sci.* 2003 Dec;1009:196-201.

818   Aricioglu F, Yillar O, Korcegez E, Berkman K. Effect of harmane on the convulsive threshold in epilepsy models in mice. *Ann N Y Acad Sci.* 2003 Dec;1009:190-5.

819   Louis ED, Benito-León J, Moreno-García S, et al. Blood harmane (1-methyl-9H-pyrido[3,4-b]indole) concentration in essential tremor cases in Spain. *Neurotoxicology.* 2013 Jan;34:264-8. doi: 10.1016/j.neuro.2012.09.004.

820   Nasehi M, Piri M, Nouri M, Farzin D, Nayer-Nouri T, Zarrindast MR. Involvement of dopamine D1/D2 receptors on harmane-induced amnesia in the step-down passive avoidance test. *Eur J Pharmacol.* 2010 May 25;634(1-3):77-83. doi: 10.1016/j.ejphar.2010.02.027.

821   Smith KL, Ford GK, Jessop DS, Finn DP. Behavioural, neurochemical and neuroendocrine effects of the endogenous β-carboline harmane in fear-conditioned rats. *J Psychopharmacol.* 2013 Feb;27(2):162-70. doi: 10.1177/0269881112460108.

822   Celikyurt IK, Utkan T, Gocmez SS, Hudson A, Aricioglu F. Effect of harmane, an endogenous β-carboline, on learning and memory in rats. *Pharmacol Biochem Behav.* 2013 Jan;103(3):666-71. doi: 10.1016/j.pbb.2012.10.011.

823   Nasehi M, Piri M, Nouri M, Farzin D, Nayer-Nouri T, Zarrindast MR. Involvement of dopamine D1/D2 receptors on harmane-induced amnesia in the step-down passive avoidance test. *Eur J Pharmacol.* 2010 May 25;634(1-3):77-83. doi: 10.1016/j.ejphar.2010.02.027.

824   Farzin D, Mansouri N. Antidepressant-like effect of harmane and other beta-carbolines in the mouse forced swim test. *Eur Neuropsychopharmacol.* 2006 Jul;16(5):324-8.

825   Tabach R, Rodrigues E, Carlini EA. Preclinical toxicological assessment of a phytotherapeutic product--CPV (based on dry extracts of Crataegus oxyacantha L., Passiflora incarnata L., and Valeriana officinalis L.). *Phytother Res.* 2009 Jan;23(1):33-40. doi: 10.1002/ptr.2499.

826   Dhawan K, Sharma A. Antitussive activity of the methanol extract of Passiflora incarnata leaves. *Fitoterapia.* 2002 Aug;73(5):397-9.

827   Breivogel C, Jamerson B. Passion flower extract antagonizes the expression of nicotine locomotor sensitization in rats. *Pharm Biol.* 2012 Oct;50(10):1310-6. doi: 10.3109/13880209.2012.674535.

828   Dhawan K, Sharma A. Antitussive activity of the methanol extract of Passiflora incarnata leaves. *Fitoterapia.* 2002 Aug;73(5):397-9.

829   Carrasco MC, Vallejo JR, Pardo-de-Santayana M, Peral D, Martín MA, Altimiras J. Interactions of Valeriana officinalis L. and Passiflora incarnata L. in a patient treated with lorazepam. *Phytother Res.* 2009 Dec;23(12):1795-6. doi: 10.1002/ptr.2847.

830   Fisher AA, Purcell P, Le Couteur DG. Toxicity of Passiflora incarnata L. *J Toxicol Clin Toxicol.* 2000;38(1):63-6.

Notes

Appendix

831   Holick MF. Resurrection of vitamin D deficiency and rickets. *J Clin Invest.* 2006 Aug;116(8):2062-72.

832   Hirayama S, Masuda Y, Rabeler R. Effect of phosphatidylserine administration on symptoms of attention-deficit/hyperactivity disorder in children. *Agro Food.* 2006;17(5):32-36.

833   Evcimen H, Mania I, Mathews M, Basil B. Psychosis Precipitated by Acetyl-l-Carnitine in a Patient with Bipolar Disorder. *Prim Care Companion J Clin Psychiatry.* 2007; 9(1): 71-72.

834   Centella asiatica. *Altern Med Rev.* 2007 Mar;12(1):69-72.

835   Mathew J, Balakrishnan S, Antony S, Abraham PM, Paulose CS. Decreased GABA receptor in the cerebral cortex of epileptic rats: effect of Bacopa monnieri and Bacoside-A. *J Biomed Sci.* 2012 Feb 24;19:25. doi: 10.1186/1423-0127-19-25.

Index

www.ingramcontent.com/pod-product-compliance
Lightning Source LLC
Chambersburg PA
CBHW060313030426
42336CB00011B/1028